# Mediterranean Diet
## 2 in 1 Box Set

*A Comprehensive Guide to the Mediterranean Diet-155 Mouth-Watering and Healthy Recipes to Help You Lose Weight, Increase Your Energy Level and Prevent Disease*

© **Copyright 2015 by Vanessa Olsen - All rights reserved.**

This document is geared towards providing exact and reliable information in regards to the topic and issue covered. The publication is sold with the idea that the publisher is not required to render accounting, officially permitted, or otherwise, qualified services. If advice is necessary, legal or professional, a practiced individual in the profession should be ordered.

- From a Declaration of Principles which was accepted and approved equally by a Committee of the American Bar Association and a Committee of Publishers and Associations.

In no way is it legal to reproduce, duplicate, or transmit any part of this document in either electronic means or in printed format. Recording of this publication is strictly prohibited and any storage of this document is not allowed unless with written permission from the publisher. All rights reserved.

The information provided herein is stated to be truthful and consistent, in that any liability, in terms of inattention or otherwise, by any usage or abuse of any policies, processes, or directions contained within is the solitary and utter responsibility of the recipient reader. Under no circumstances will any legal responsibility or blame be held against the publisher for any reparation, damages, or monetary loss due to the information herein, either directly or indirectly.

Respective authors own all copyrights not held by the publisher.

The information herein is offered for informational purposes solely, and is universal as so. The presentation of the information is without contract or any type of guarantee assurance.

The trademarks that are used are without any consent, and the publication of the trademark is without permission or backing by the trademark owner. All trademarks and brands within this book are for clarifying purposes only and are the owned by the owners themselves, not affiliated with this document.

# MEDITERRANEAN DIET

## 50 Amazing Recipes for Weight Loss and Improved Health

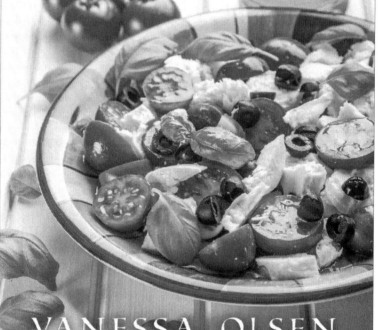

### VANESSA OLSEN

# Table of Contents

Introduction

Chapter 1: Up until Now

Chapter 2: The Good Stuff

Chapter 3: What You'll Be Eating

Chapter 4: Tips for Success

Chapter 5: 50 Scrumptious Recipes

### BREAKFAST

- Omelet Muffins
- Good Morning Couscous
- Mediterranean Hash Browns
- Green Eggs and Toast
- Fluffy Mediterranean Pancakes
- Fruity Yoghurt Parfait
- Spanish Omelet
- Classic Breakfast Sandwich
- Mediterranean Egg-in-the-Hole
- Chicken and Veggie Breakfast Wraps

### LUNCH

- Seafood Pasta
- An Elegant Lady's Pizza
- Spicy Pita Burgers
- Greek-Style Couscous
- Classic Greek Salad
- Mediterranean Pasta Salad
- Mediterranean Shish Kebabs
- Greek-Approved Fried Rice
- Spanish Tuna Melts
- Classic Submarine Sandwich

### DINNER

- Salmon with all the Fixings
- Chickpea Burgers
- Stuffed Portobello Mushrooms
- Cheesy Eggplant Sandwiches
- Vegetarian Pasta Bolognese
- Spanish Seafood Fried Rice
- Chicken with Greek-Style Quinoa Salad
- Italian Potato Salad
- Roasted Veggies
- Breadcrumbs for Dinner

## SNACKS

- Feta Cheese and Olives Marinade
- Tomato Tea Party Sandwiches
- Dates in a Blanket
- Veggie Shish Kebabs
- Mediterranean Sushi
- Roasted Chickpeas
- Sweet-Baked Banana
- Spicy Red Pepper Spread
- Tomato Poached Mozzarella Balls
- Mini Shrimp Cakes

## DESSERT

- Grilled Peaches and Cream
- Toasted Sesame Ganache
- Warm, sweet, hot cherries
- Walnut Spice Bars
- Nutty Banana Bread
- Greek Almond Cake
- Pistachio Batter Cake
- Chia Chocolate Balls
- Simple Gelato
- Peanut Butter Chocolate Chip Cookies

Chapter 6: 7 Days of Food

Chapter 7: Adjusting the Meal Plan

Chapter 8: Mediterranean Myths

Epilogue

# Introduction

Too many times I see it happen. People go on diets with high hopes of a better life or finally achieving the body of their dreams only to give up a couple of weeks in. What happens to all the dreaming and strong spirits? Truth be told, it's usually the fault of the diet.

Too many diets are built around strict guidelines and nutrient counts which are far too low. They make us sluggish, hungry, and irritable within a couple days. Think of it this way: your body runs on food, and so food runs your life. Feed yourself well and your body will do you well. Feed yourself poorly and it should go without saying your body won't be capable of much.

The Mediterranean diet, in contrast, is different from all others existing today. There are no strict rules, no foods which are completely off limits, and no lack in nutrients. The Mediterranean diet is about creating a healthy lifestyle as have the people in the Mediterranean region. It's based on tradition from the crops to the ocean to the dinner table in the way the Mediterranean people harvest, fish, conserve, process, and prepare their foods. The Mediterranean is actually not a diet as the name would have you believe – it's simply a way of life.

The Mediterranean diet is based on simple foods that are brought to life with imagination and the right spices. Its broad range of possibilities offers people all the advantages of a healthy diet linked to the land of origin. It incorporates the customs the lively people of the Mediterranean basin have based their lives off of for generations. It is a choice which is tried, tested, logical, and simple. It is a choice which could finally change your life in the way you've been hoping for a long time now.

In the next pages you will be provided with a deep look into the history of the Mediterranean diet, a lengthy list of the benefits it will bring to your life, information on how you yourself should go about following it, myths associated with the diet, and tips for success. As the title of this book promises, you will also find 50 deliciously simple tried and tested recipes along with an adjustable 7 day meal plan to get you started. I believe that anyone who puts in the effort deserves to feel happy and fulfilled, and I'm so excited to see how this guide on one of the most successful diets in history will do just that for you.

# Chapter 1 – Up until Now

The Mediterranean diet is, as you've probably guessed based on the name, a diet based on foods historically eaten in the Mediterranean region. It is here that the entirety of the ancient world's history unfolded itself, and the place historians refer to as "the cradle of society".

This chapter will show how the Mediterranean diet came together, bit by bit, in chronological order. It's quite interesting to see how exploring new worlds and experiencing different cultures shaped the Mediterranean diet into the form we know it as today.

753 BC – 476 AD: The Mediterranean diet began with the Ancient Romans and Egyptians. Information is surprisingly abundant on these origins. Archeologists have found the diet documented through the likes of art, tools, pottery, inscription on stone, and in rare cases, food debris. The biggest source of evidence, however, is through the works of ancient authors from the time period. It is through literary works that scholars can conclude there was an impressively large variety of food and drinks available to the Romans in this time. And not only was this smorgasbord prepared in different ways, but it was enjoyed in different ways as well – whether at a casual meal or banquet.

By examining this evidence, it is apparent that the wealthy indulged mostly in breads, oils, and wines. They also had sheep cheese and vegetables such as mushrooms, lettuce, chicory, mallow, and leeks but only ate these foods in smaller amounts because at the time, they were "... considered beneath the dignity of gods and heroes". Very tiny amounts of meat could also be found scattered in their diet, while fish and seafood was available, again, only to the wealthiest classes. Slaves were obviously less fortunate, having a monthly allowance of bread, a half-pound of olives, olive oil, and salted fish. Rarely were they also given meat, but they were very grateful when they were.

It was during this time period that the Germans and Romans clashed, introducing the likes of pork and grains in the form of beer. These introductions were temporary, however, as the Romans decided to remain firm in their original diet mostly composed of bread, oil, and wine.

After the clash of the Germans and the Romans was when the Arabians began to add to the Mediterranean diet. They brought about foods like sugar, spice, rice, spinach, eggplant, pomegranate, rose water, almonds, lemons, and oranges. This added the element of variety which is a defining feature of the Mediterranean diet today.

1492: The model of the Mediterranean diet remained untouched for generations until Christopher Columbus made the courageous voyage into new worlds and discovered America. This discovery of course sparked a mixing of many different cultures and traditions, but mostly in food. The Mediterranean diet now included American foods such as potatoes, beans, peppers, corn, chili, and tomatoes. The tomato, in particular, became a symbol for the Mediterranean diet, as it stood out against all other plant foods involved.

Secondary to the introduction of the tomato was the introduction of cereals. No, I'm not referring to cereals along the lines of Lucky Charms or Honey Nut Cheerios, but rather anything from bread to pasta to couscous to polenta. These cereals carried a lot of importance during this time in America, as they held a strong "ability to fill" and kept the poorer classes alive in times of struggle.

1948: The first known attempt to research the Mediterranean diet in depth was after World War 2. At the time, the government of Greece was desperate to improve their country's postwar conditions. From economic to social to health, they knew there was a lot of fixing up to do. So, they invited the Rockerfeller Foundation to figure out a way to best raise their people's standard of living by conducting an epidemiologic study on the island of Crete. The Rockerfeller

Foundation chose epidemiologist, Leland Allbaugh, to take on the job. Allbaugh determinedly rose to the challenge, examining the demographic, dietary, economic, social, and health characteristic of 1 of every 150 random households on the island. The results can be seen in the table below.

| | Greece: food balance 1948-1949 | Crete: 7-d diet Record | Household inventory[2] |
|---|---|---|---|
| Energy | | | |
| (MJ/d) | 10.2 | 10.6 | 10.7 |
| (kcal/d) | 2443 | 2547 | 2554 |
| Foods (kg · person[-1] · y[-1]) | | | |
| Cereals | 158.2 | 127.7 | 128.2 |
| Potatoes | 30.9 | 59.1 | 38.6 |
| Sugar and honey | 9.1 | 5.5 | 5.5 |
| Pulses and nuts | 15.0 | 20.0 | 23.2 |
| Vegetables, fruits, and | | | |
| Olives | 120.5 | 175.9 | 132.3 |
| Meat, fish, and eggs | 23.2 | 28.6 | 27.7 |
| Milk and cheese | 35.0 | 25.5 | 34.5 |
| Oils and fats | 15.0 | 30.9 | 30.9 |
| Wine, beer, and spirits | 37.7 | 10.0 | 38.6 |

At the end of the study, Allbaugh found that although the diet of the Crete people was nutritionally adequate to US standards, the people of Crete were often hungry finding that the diet did not fulfill their nutritional needs. He concluded that their diet could be improved by adding more meat, cheese, fish, butter, and pasta.

1950s: In an effort to address the epidemic of cardiovascular disease in Western society, American scientist of the University Of Minnesota School Of Power, Ancel Keys, did some research regarding the relationship food had with the disease. Keys noticed that the health of people living in Italy's poorest towns was better than the health of the wealthiest people living in New York City, and wanted to find out why. Upon travelling to Italy and visiting these poor towns, he found that they ate a diet consisting mostly of homemade pasta noodles covered in tomato sauce and sprinkled with cheese. Sometimes they would add meat or seafood to their pasta, but only a couple times a week. Besides pasta, they also ate beans, fresh-baked bread, lots of veggies, and fruit for dessert. Wine was often the drink to accompany adult meals. Keys took note that this diet was incredibly low in fat and half the size of a standard American meal. With these factors in mind, Keys concluded that there was no better diet to prevent cardiovascular disease than the diet of the Italians, especially when compared to the American diet far too rich in meat and dairy.

1960s: Pleased with his findings after examining the Italian diet, Keys hired a team of colleagues in order to expand the study. This expansion was called the "Seven Countries Study", which closely examined the lifestyles of 13,000 middle-aged men living in Finland, Holland, Italy, United States, Greece, Japan, and Yugoslavia.

1989: Keys published the results of the Seven Countries Study. The report shows the effects that different intakes of bread, cereal, alcohol, fat, sweets, vegetables, fruit, eggs, meat, dairy, and fish has on cholesterol and cardiovascular disease. These data also showed that the Mediterranean diet had changed a bit since ancient times. The Mediterranean diet of the 1960's was now mostly comprised of plant foods, with some versions, thanks to olive oil, being higher in fat than others. The versions higher in fat showed to support a population of overall healthier people than versions lower in fat. Keys found there was a strong connection between overall health and the intake of good fats, noting that people eating a "Mediterranean diet" were much healthier overall than those on other diets.

1990s – Present Day: Keys' observations have become much more widely known, and the Mediterranean diet has gained lots of credibility for the benefits it produces. As a result, many more studies have been conducted on the effects that the Mediterranean diet has on cardiovascular health and chronic illness; with almost every single one concluding the effects are positive. Additionally, the diet also shows it benefits those who are suffering from obesity, high blood sugar and triglyceride levels, and low density lipoprotein. Needless to say, jumping onto the Mediterranean bandwagon has become a standard practice for those who wish to better their health in today's world.

# Chapter 2 – The Good Stuff

Although we've already touched briefly on this topic in the last chapter, I've decided to lay the benefits of the Mediterranean diet out in more depth since they are seemingly bottomless. Whether it's something you are trying to prevent or something you are trying to cure – the Mediterranean diet is there for you.

Cardiovascular disease – The Mediterranean diet encourages foods like whole grains, seafood, and red wine instead of refined breads, red meat, and hard liquor which are all culprits for causing cardiovascular disease. In fact, research has found that the Mediterranean diet is far more effective than a low-fat diet in preventing the development of cardiovascular disease. Those who adhere to the guidelines of the Mediterranean diet are actually 30% less likely to develop cardiovascular disease than those who don't. It has also showed to lower levels of bad cholesterol in the blood while increasing levels of good cholesterol in the blood.

Stroke – A recent PREDIMED study as published by the New England Journal of Medicine shows that following a Mediterranean diet results in a 30% reduction in stroke among those with serious cardiovascular illness. In addition, chair of neurology at North Shore University Hospital has stated that properly following the guidelines of the Mediterranean diet significantly reduces the chance of ischemic stroke caused by blood clot.

Type 2 Diabetes – Research from the UK shows that those living with type 2 diabetes can reap the most benefits on a Mediterranean diet than they can on a vegetarian, vegan, low-carb, high-protein, or high-fiber diet. Additionally, more than 5 major studies show that the Mediterranean diet substantially lowers the risk of developing type 2 diabetes in people of all sorts (healthy and unhealthy). Studies have also shown that a Mediterranean diet will help those with type 2 diabetes better control glycemic levels and achieve cardiovascular benefits as foods associated with the diet are high in polyphenols. Some extremely important added benefits include weight loss and lower cholesterol levels.

High blood pressure – This illness is responsible for one in every three deaths that occur in the USA. A Mediterranean diet can help prevent the development of high blood pressure as it is rich in potassium, calcium, and magnesium while being low in sodium. This is thanks to the fact that the diet is based on foods such as fruits, vegetables, and olive oil.

Alzheimer's – While it is unclear exactly how the Mediterranean diet preserves brain function, extensive research does show it has reverse effects on Alzheimer's disease. Research has proven it can slow mental decline that comes with age, reduce the risk of mild cognitive impairment, reduce the risk of mild cognitive impairment turning into Alzheimer's, and slow the general progression of Alzheimer's disease. It is speculated that these effects are possible thanks to the healthy food choices which improve levels of cholesterol, blood sugar, and overall blood vessel health, in turn reducing the risk of Alzheimer's.

Cancer – Research published in the British Journal of Cancer states that replacing bad fats with good fats and eating more vegetables as opposed to meat can cut risk of developing cancer by 12%. In fact, a study conducted by professor of cancer prevention and epidemiology at Harvard University took a look at 26,000 Greek men and women over the period of 8 years to find that "... those who closely followed a traditional Mediterranean diet were overall less likely to develop cancer".

Parkinson's – A solid link between the Mediterranean diet and prevention of Parkinson's disease is yet to be determined. However, researchers have determined that those who more closely follow a Mediterranean style diet in their lifetime have lower chances of developing Parkinson's disease. The researchers who conducted this study stated that "lower

Mediterranean-type diet score was associated with earlier Parkinson's disease age at onset." Researchers speculate that Parkinson's disease could be prevented by the Mediterranean diet because the diet involves food lower in compounds which are associated with Parkinson's disease. The Mediterranean diet has also showed to reduce oxidative stress and inflammation, which are factors known to cause Parkinson's.

Obesity – Many people jump the Mediterranean diet bandwagon to lose weight... and for good reason! According to the journal Obesity Reviews, those who go on the Mediterranean diet while at a healthy weight have less chance of becoming obese, and according to a study published in The Journal of the American Medical Association, those who go on the diet while overweight are likely to shed some extra pounds. These statements are especially true when the diet is used in conjunction with exercise.

Agility – The food involved with the Mediterranean diet is jam packed with nutrients known to keep us strong, fit, and healthy for life! In fact, those who adhere to the diet's specifications until old age are 70% less likely to have their muscles go limp or experience other sides of frailty as is common with old age.

Longevity – Not only does the Mediterranean diet help to keep us strong, fit, and healthy until old age, but it can also ensure we live longer too! Researchers say that the Mediterranean diet will actually reduce the risk of death at any age by 20%.

Mind – As it turns out, the Mediterranean diet is beneficial in ways other than physical. A study conducted by the University of Las Palmas de Gran Canaria and the University of Navarra looked at a group of 11,000 students for four years. A quality of life evaluation was taken at the beginning of the study and at the end, after 4 years. By the end of the 4 years, the results showed that those who stuck to the Mediterranean diet reported to have both a better quality of life and wellbeing.

So there you have it, folks. Whether you're going Mediterranean to beat or prevent a chronic illness, lose weight, or just improve your quality of life in general, you've come to the right place. When we think of the people in the Mediterranean region, we think of people full of love, life, and compassion, and that's exactly what the Mediterranean diet could bring about for you.

# Chapter 3 – What You'll Be Eating

After reading about the benefits the Mediterranean diet is capable of, you're probably interested in knowing more about exactly how it works. In particular, what exactly you will be eating. Well, it all depends on how much physical activity you do or how many calories you burn each day. However, there is a model which anyone can follow, no matter how much exercise they do, that will still lead them to their goals of health and weight loss. Let me break it down for you…

The nutrient you will be consuming the most of is carbs. Many people are put off by this, as there is a notion out there that the less carbs you eat the more weight you will lose. However, you may be surprised to learn that for the most part, this notion is far from true. In fact, eating a diet full of the right sorts of carbs will help you lose weight, build muscle, keep your energy levels up, make you feel more full, and spark your metabolism. While on the Mediterranean diet, 55-60% of your calories will come from carbs, with a whopping 80% of these carbs being "complex". Not sure what a complex carb is? No problem, you can use this handy list as reference.

| | | |
|---|---|---|
| Spinach | Whole Barley | Grapefruit |
| Turnip Greens | Buckwheat | Apples |
| Lettuce | Buckwheat bread | Prunes |
| Water Cress | Oat bran bread | Apricots, Dried |
| Zucchini | Oatmeal | Pears |
| Asparagus | Oat bran cereal | Plums |
| Artichokes | Museli | Strawberries |
| Okra | Wild rice | Oranges |
| Cabbage | Brown rice | Yams |
| Celery | Multi-grain bread | Carrots |
| Cucumbers | Pinto beans | Potatoes |
| Dill Pickles | Yogurt low fat | Soybeans |
| Radishes | Skim milk | Lentils |
| Broccoli | Navy beans | Garbanzo beans |
| Brussels Sprouts | Cauliflower | Kidney beans |
| Eggplant | Soy milk | Lentils |
| Onions | Whole meal spelt bread | Split peas |
| Tomatoes | | |

The next most dominant nutrient in the Mediterranean diet is fat. Have I got your head spinning yet? You must be thinking, "Carbs AND fat and I'm going to lose weight/get healthier?" And the answer is yes! Both of those things will happen for you, as long as you eat the right fat. So, 25-30% of your calories will come from fat, with at least 80% of this fat coming from olive oil. Yes, as you read in the Up Until Now chapter, the people of the Mediterranean region just LOVED their olive oil, and you're going to as well.

The smallest main nutrient of the Mediterranean diet is protein – 15-20%% of your calories intake, to be exact. 60% of these proteins will come from animals, especially fish, chicken, and rabbit. Red meat is to be consumed only on rare occasions, about once a month.

Other foods to eat in smaller quantities include fruit and red wine. Those of the Mediterranean region have always paired meals with red wine and finished them off with a healthy bowl of fruit. Health practitioners say women should drink one glass of wine per day, men one to two, accompanied by two servings of fresh fruit.

So, now that you have all the calorie percentages, you may be wondering exactly how many calories you will be basing these percentages off of. This will depend on a few factors, but there is software online to take the math out of it and give you an exact number. My favorite is **Calorie King**. They take into consideration your height, weight, age, gender, and activity levels to give you the most accurate range of calories you should consume daily. Then, you choose whether you are looking to lose, gain, or maintain your current weight and Calorie King give you a number tailored to that goal.

Go to Calorie King at:
http://www.calorieking.com/interactive-tools/how-many-calories-should-you-eat/

Once you know how many calories you should be consuming per day, you can do the math to see exactly how much of what nutrient you should be eating on the Mediterranean diet. The math will look something like this:

a = your daily calorie intake
b = amount of daily calories which should come from said nutrient

*Carbs:*
a x 0.55 = b
a x 0.60 = b
*Fat:*
a x 0.25 = b
a x 0.30 = b
*Protein:*
a x 0.15 = b
a x 0.20 = b

If algebra isn't your strongest suit (and believe me, it isn't mine either), let me show you a real life example. Calorie King says that my optimal daily calorie intake should be between 1,600-1,800 calories per day. Matching the low end of my calorie range with the lower percentage and the high end of my calorie intake with the higher percentage, this is how the math looks.

*Carbs:*
1,600 x 0.55 = 880
1,800 x 0.60 = 1080
This means that 880-1,080 of my daily calories should come from sources high in carbs.

*Fat:*
1,600 x 0.25 = 400
1,800 x 0.30 = 540
This means that 400-540 of my daily calories should come from sources high in fat, specifically olive oil.

*Protein:*
1,600 x 0.15 = 240
1,800 x 0.20 = 360

This means that 240-360 of my daily calories should come from sources high in protein.

Foods to completely avoid while on the Mediterranean diet include sweet foods, soda pop, processed foods, and fast foods. You didn't see the ancient Romans devouring those sorts of things, so you won't either!

It's important to remember that adopting the Mediterranean diet doesn't only entail you adopt changes in your diet. Things like exercise and socializing are important as well – it's part of the Mediterranean way of life! Take the stairs at work and have a family sit down meal that encourages conversation. Incorporating these factors means improving your health in more areas than one. Additionally, it's important to avoid stress, smoking, and excessive drinking as these factors can slow your progress.

# Chapter 4 – Tips for Success

Making drastic lifestyle changes are never easy, but this guide was designed with the intention of making the switch to the Mediterranean diet as simple as possible. In this chapter, you will find advice on how to prepare for the smoothest transition possible and how to stay on track. This chapter will be super handy whenever you feel your motivation drop or your willpower giving in!

## Preparing to make the switch...

Thinking back –

How have you made drastic lifestyle changes in your life previously? For example, if you have quit smoking before, did you cut the habit cold turkey, or was the process more gradual? Evaluating how you've successfully made a lifestyle change before will help you decide the best way to go about incorporating the Mediterranean diet.

After reflecting –

If you noticed you're more the all-or-nothing type, raid your cupboards. Get rid of anything that is full of sugar, full of chemicals, or processed. Most of these things come in a box or package. Then, get yourself re-stocked. You can read up on some grocery shopping tips and tricks below.

If you noticed you like to take your time implementing lifestyle changes, eat what you have now. Yep, go for it! Just make sure when you go grocery shopping that you only buy food that's Mediterranean friendly. This way all that unhealthy junk will gradually make its way out of the house, giving you more time to adjust to the change.

Grocery shopping –

Whether you decided to make a sudden jump into the world of Mediterranean foods or let the change come more gradually, every trip you now make to the grocery store will revolve around finding foods which fit Mediterranean cuisine. While browsing the isles, it's important you remember to not give into foods just because they're labeled as "Mediterranean" or "healthy". More often than not, these labels lie! Instead, put your efforts into buying whole foods – the fruits, veggies, fish, and cereal grains we talked about in the What You'll Be Eating chapter. The key to a successful Mediterranean diet is having lots and lots of variety! For example, eating lots of different fruits and veggies means your body will get a very broad range of all those awesome vitamins, minerals, and nutrients. Of course, make sure that nothing which is full of sugar, full of chemicals or processed lands a spot in your buggy. Also, we people of the Western world tend to put way too much salt in our foods. The people of the Mediterranean diet instead use herbs and spices to give their food flavor, so it's a good idea to pay a visit to that isle.

With all this being said, I too know the struggle of buying unfamiliar foods and leaving old favorites behind, so be sure to check out 50 Scrumptious Recipes chapter found at the end of this book. It will show you the types of ingredients you'll need and give you a better idea of what you should buy.

Knowing your kitchen –

The Mediterranean diet is based on whole foods which require a bit of preparation. If boxed meals that require minimal kitchen-work are what you're used to, then it may be beneficial for you to get to know your kitchen a bit better before you're required to prepare Mediterranean meals from scratch. Being successful on the Mediterranean diet also means having a kitchen fully stocked with a variety of pots, pans, measuring cups, and knives. If you're a bit short on materials, a trip to the Dollar Store should fix you up! Also be sure that you're familiar with how to prep and cook a wide variety of different foods. If your skills need a bit of work, there are many cooking tutorials you can watch on YouTube for free! The best part about becoming skilled in the kitchen means having full control over the ingredients you consume and taking pride in the food you eat. It's a great feeling, to say the least.

Assemble the troops –

Some days you may encounter situations which require more will power than you're even sure you have. For example, a co-worker may set a box of donuts in the break room or a family get together may have a spread of sugar-filled treats. To help smooth these situations over, begin to scatter Mediterranean approved goodies around. I like to keep mine in my purse, desk drawer, car, or sometimes if I'm feeling extra cheeky – even in my nightstand. Having these goodies on hand will help to curb temptation as you'll have your own, more healthy, goodies on hand. I suggest trying the Toasted Sesame Ganache found in the recipes chapter. Those things are conveniently tiny and compact – slip them into a Ziploc baggy and they're good to go just about anywhere!

Kill those cravings –

Many people aren't successful in making healthy lifestyle changes because their efforts are overcome by intense cravings. In order to make sure this doesn't happen to you, it may be beneficial to start thinking of some ways to kill your bad-food cravings. Strategies usually come in the form of juice cleanses, supplements, and mental tricks and it may take a little experimentation to find out which works best for you. I'm not going to sugar-coat things for you (pun unintended!), kicking a craving is always terribly difficult at first. But trust me, if you can stick to your guns for long enough those awful cravings will soon diminish, even to the point that the food which you once craved so much won't even taste good anymore.

Know your nutrients –

As stated in the What You'll Be Eating chapter, the Mediterranean diet is broken down into a couple of main nutrients – carbs, fat, and protein. Knowing exactly how much of which you should eat will help you out tons when you first start out. That being said, don't be afraid to refer back to the What You'll Be Eating chapter over and over until you know it like the back of your hand. Getting those nutrients right is key to living the healthy Mediterranean lifestyle.

**While you're on the diet...**

Remember your fruits and veggies –

I cannot stress enough the importance veggies carry in the Mediterranean diet! There are lots of ways you can incorporate them into things you're already used to eating – you just have to be creative! For example, instead of having toast with a spread of butter and cheddar cheese you could have toast with a smattering of olive oil, crumbled feta cheese, and tomatoes. Salads, soups, and oatmeal topped with fruit are other great ways to ensure you get a sufficient amount of fruits and veggies. The trick to getting your fill is in incorporating them into meals and eating them as snacks between meals whenever possible.

Never skip a breakfast –

I remember my mother used to lecture me about how "breakfast is the most important meal of the day!" and while I'm not too keen to admit this, I have to admit that she was right. Skipping breakfast will make you hungrier later in the day, which could make you inclined to binge on a "cheat" meal. Eating a breakfast composed of fruits, whole grains, and maybe even some veggies will keep you full until lunch time, plus spark your metabolism for the day. Your future self with thank you!

Fish is a friend –

Try to get some seafood into your diet twice a week. The Mediterranean's ate lots of seafood rich in healthy Omega-3 fatty acids such as tuna, clams, salmon, oysters, herring, mussels, and sardines. Those who suffer from cardiovascular disease will especially benefit from a diet containing modest amounts of seafood.

Go vegetarian every once in a while –

Health practitioners suggest that those on the Mediterranean diet boycott meat for one day of the week. Simply choose a day and dedicate it to creating meals based on beans, whole grains, and vegetables. If you begin to get the feeling you're getting a hang of vegetarian cooking, aim to go vegetarian for two nights a week. The more the merrier, as meats should be eaten sparingly.

Load up on healthy fats –

Stop fearing healthy fats just because they have the word "fat" in them! Foods like extra-virgin olive oil, avocados, nuts, olives, and sunflower seeds are full of these healthy fats known to nourish your body in ways which no other nutrient can. As you introduce more and more good fats to your diet, be sure to eliminate the bad ones as well. Fat sources which aren't doing you any favors include margarine, butter, vegetable shortening, cookies, French fries, and potato chips, to name a few.

Start substituting –

When making the change to a healthier lifestyle, it may be difficult to cut foods out cold-turkey. This method makes us feel like something is missing, meaning we'll be more inclined to go back to our old ways. Instead, try replacing unhealthy foods with healthier alternatives, and make mental note of these substitutions. For example, animal fats can be replaced with vegetable fats. A slice of avocado or tomato can be used on your toast instead of cheese. Snacking on cookies can be traded for snacking on olives, nuts, or veggies. And your tall glass of beer at dinner can be replaced with a glass of red wine. The theory is that you won't miss the old food as much if you have a new, healthier alternative to put in its place.

Read ingredient lists –

As mentioned, just because manufacturers label foods as "healthy" or "Mediterranean" it doesn't exactly mean their product lives up to those standards. If you do want to buy packaged foods, you need to know how to read labels. An ingredients list which mentions anything along the lines of added sugar, salt, chemicals, or preservatives means the product is far from healthy and should be left on the shelf.

Plan big, eat small –

When Ancel Keys went to Italy to study the Mediterranean diet, he took notice that their portion sizes were considerably smaller than those typical in the Western world. And it's true – serving sizes here are much bigger than necessary. If you're eating a meal packed with all the right nutrients, vitamins, and minerals, you shouldn't need to eat such copious amounts of food. When you're preparing a meal, try choosing visual cues to keep your portion sizes under control. For example, a serving of chicken, meat, or seafood the size of a deck of cards is sufficient for one meal. Whole grains such as brown rice, pasta, and oats eaten in a portion size similar to a light bulb will do as well. If in the beginning you feel it's tricky sticking to these portion sizes, add more greens to your meal or have some fruit for dessert.

Chew before you swallow –

Taking time to eat food is a factor of a healthy diet that's often overlooked. It will usually take a few minutes for your stomach to tell your brain that it's full, so chew your food thoroughly and savor the flavors. Eating too quickly can lead to eating more than is necessary.

Enjoy your food with others –

This tip is more encouraged in the Mediterranean diet than any other. The people of the Mediterranean region saw meal time as a way to connect and enjoy the company of those around them – and you should too! Not only does it promote emotional benefits and healthy eating, but it also prevents mindless overeating that happens when dining in front of the TV.

The night is for sleeping –

Avoid eating too late at night while on the Mediterranean diet. Meals which are eaten too close to bedtime are usually stored as excess fat since your body doesn't burn it off. Instead, have an early dinner and then try to fast for 14-15 hours until breakfast the next morning. For example, if you have a 7AM wake up, try to eat your dinner around 4-5PM the evening previous. This allows your digestive system to take a long break which studies suggest can help regulate weight.

**Keeping it going...**

Take notes –

How are you feeling, doing, progressing? In particular, how do you feel once you're done with a meal? You should feel a little healthier and better about yourself each time. Taking note of this will help you to love your new lifestyle even more, and keep you away from going back to your old ways which only left you feeling unhealthy and sluggish.

When things seem too difficult –

Make them simpler! For many, the process of counting nutrients can be a little tiresome. If you feel that counting calories is actually slowing your progress, then instead simply focus your energy on making sure you're getting lots of variety, color, and fresh foods. This could be named as the rule of thumb for any clean-eating diet, but especially the Mediterranean.

The power of your mind –

An anonymous source once quoted that "We are never satisfied with what we have. We want what we can't have and take the things we do have for granted". This logic applies to dieting as well. Usually, when we put it in our heads that we absolutely cannot eat something, it only makes us want to eat it more. Instead, remind yourself that you most definitely can have that treat, it is in fact 100% possible for you to eat and digest it, but your desire to feel healthy and revitalized is stronger. This way of thinking will help make cravings less intense.

# Chapter 5 – 50 Scrumptious Recipes

As promised, here are those 50 recipes! Included are 10 breakfasts, 10 lunches, 10 dinners, 10 snacks, and 10 desserts to ensure everyone will be able to eat the Mediterranean way and enjoy it too! Food is meant to be celebrated, and that's exactly what I hope these recipes turn your dinners into – whether it's a lonesome Tuesday night or a happening Saturday.


## BREAKFAST

### Omelet Muffins (makes 6 muffins)

Ingredients:
6 slices deli ham, cut thick
8 egg whites
1 egg
1 large sweet pepper, roasted
1/3 cup spinach, finely chopped
¼ cup low fat feta, broken in tiny pieces
1 ½ tablespoons pesto
Dash of pepper
Basil to garnish

Directions:
1. Preheat oven to 400 degrees Fahrenheit.
2. Rub olive oil over a muffin tin with 6 hollows.
3. Wrap a slice of ham around the inner circumference of each muffin hollow.
4. Peel black skin off roasted pepper.
5. Slice pepper into 12 pieces.
6. Put one slice of pepper into each muffin hollow, laying it on the bottom surface.
7. Sprinkle about 1 tablespoon of spinach into each muffin hollow.
8. Sprinkle a generous ½ tablespoon of feta cheese into each muffin hollow.

9. Mix together egg whites, whole egg, and pepper in a bowl.
10. Pour mixture, divided evenly, into each muffin hollow.
11. Place muffin tin in oven. Let bake for about 16 minutes or until eggs are cooked.
12. Once egg is cooked, remove the muffin tin from the oven.
13. With a baking spatula, carefully remove the omelet muffins from their hollows.
14. Garnish with leftover pepper slices, pesto and basil.
15. Plate and enjoy!

Nutritional Information (per one muffin):
Calories – 106
Fat in grams – 5
Carbs in grams – 3
Fiber in grams – 0
Protein in grams – 13

**Good Morning Couscous (makes 2 servings)**

Ingredients:
1 ½ cups milk, low-fat variety
½ cup whole-grain couscous, raw
¼ cup dried apricots, diced
2 tablespoons dried currants
3 teaspoons brown sugar
1 inch cinnamon stick

Directions:
1. Place a medium saucepan with milk and cinnamon stick over medium-high heat. Take off when small bubbles begin to form around the pan's edges – be careful not to boil!
2. Remove from heat.
3. Add couscous, apricots, 2 teaspoons brown sugar, and dried currants. Stir until well incorporated.
4. Cover pan and let mixture sit for 13-15 minutes, or until couscous has cooked.

5. Uncover and take the cinnamon stick out.
6. Top with butter and remaining brown sugar, portion into two bowls, and enjoy!

Nutritional Information (per one serving):
Calories - 306
Fat in grams – 6
Carbs in grams – 55
Fiber in grams – 5
Protein in grams – 11

## Mediterranean Hash Browns (makes 4 servings)

Ingredients:
2 cups freezer brand hash browns
7 ounces chickpeas, cleaned
1 cup baby spinach, minced
½ cup zucchini, diced
½ cup olive oil
¼ cup onion, minced
2 eggs
½ tablespoon curry powder
½ tablespoon ginger, minced

Directions:
1. In a medium bowl, mix hash browns, spinach, onion, curry powder, and ginger until well incorporated.
2. Place a (preferably nonstick) skillet with olive oil over stove on medium-high heat.
3. Scoop hash brown mixture into skillet. Form an even, compressed layer.
4. Let sit 2-4 minutes, or until the bottom is crispy and starting to brown.
5. Turn heat down to medium low.
6. Incorporate chickpeas and zucchini by breaking up chunks of hash brown until roughly combined.
7. Again, form an even, compressed layer.
8. With a wooden spoon, dig out two holes, evenly spaced, in the hash brown mixture.

9. Crack eggs into a bowl and whisk until bubbly. Evenly divide into the holes in the hash brown mixture.
10. Continue to cook for about 3-4 minutes, or until yolk have cooked.
11. Remove from skillet, slice into 4 pieces, and enjoy!

Nutritional Information (per serving):
Calories – 479
Fat in grams – 40
Carbs in grams – 25
Fiber in grams – 3
Protein in grams – 8

## Green Eggs and Toast (makes 1 serving)

Ingredients:
1 avocado, skin and pit removed
2 slices whole grain bread
2 eggs, cooked to preference
1 ½ ounces feta, broken into tiny pieces
1 tablespoon mint, minced
½ tablespoon lemon juice
Dash of pepper
Dash of lemon juice

Directions:
1. Mash avocado in a bowl using a potato masher or fork. Mix in mint, pepper, and lemon juice until well combined.
2. Toast bread to your preference.
3. Once bread has toasted, spread on the avocado mixture, dividing evenly between slices of toast.
4. Place egg cooked to your preference on top.
5. Sprinkle feta cheese and pepper overtop.
6. Plate and enjoy!

Nutritional Information (per one serving):
Calories – 604
Fat in grams – 52
Carbs in grams – 59

Fiber in grams – 24
Protein in grams – 33

## Fluffy Mediterranean Pancakes (makes 10 pancakes)

Ingredients:
¾ cup yoghurt, low-fat
½ cup whole wheat pancake mix
½ cup strawberries, stem removed and diced
1/3 cup milk, fat-free
1 egg, small
2 tablespoons olive oil
1 tablespoon maple syrup

Directions:
1. In a bowl, whisk together yoghurt, milk, and egg until bubbly.
2. Bit by bit, stir in whole wheat pancake mix.
3. Put a pan with a bit of the olive oil over medium-high heat.
4. Portioning mixture evenly, fry 10 pancakes. They should take about 2-3 minutes each side.
5. Serve, topping with strawberries and maple syrup.
6. Enjoy!

Nutrient Breakdown (per 1 pancake):
Calories – 143
Fat in grams – 4
Carbs in grams – 17
Fiber in grams – 1
Protein in grams – 6

## Fruity Yoghurt Parfait (makes 2 parfaits)

Ingredients:
12 ounces yoghurt, low-fat
2 cups raspberries
4 tablespoons granola, low-fat

Directions:

1. Assemble ingredients and have two wide-mouth glasses in front of you.
2. Layer the ingredients in the glasses, starting with yoghurt, then raspberries, and repeat.
3. Once you're out of yoghurt and raspberries, top each parfait with 2 tablespoons granola
4. Serve with a long spoon and enjoy!

Nutrient Breakdown (per one parfait):
Calories – 222
Fat in grams – 4
Carbs in grams – 36
Fiber in grams – 9
Protein in grams – 12

**Spanish Omelet (makes 2 servings)**

Ingredients:
4 eggs
1 ounce goat cheese
¼ cup milk, low-fat
½ tomato, diced
1 tablespoon chives, chopped
1 teaspoon olive oil
Dash of pepper

Directions:
1. Heat oven to 375 degrees Fahrenheit.
2. Whisk together eggs, milk, and pepper, in a medium sized bowl until bubbles form.
3. Once bubbles have formed, incorporate tomato and chives.
4. Put a skillet with the olive oil over stove on medium heat.
5. Once skillet is hot, pour in egg mixture.
6. Bit by bit, crumble goat cheese into skillet.
7. Cook goat cheese and egg mixture for 2-3 minutes, or until egg around edges is cooked.

8. Put the skillet in the oven and let sit for 8-9 minutes or until egg has cooked through.
9. Plate and enjoy with fresh fruit!

Nutritional Breakdown (per serving):
Calories – 222
Fat in grams – 16
Carbs in grams – 4
Fiber in grams – 0
Protein in grams – 17

## Classic Breakfast Sandwich (makes 1 serving)

Ingredients:
1 multigrain English muffin
1 cup baby spinach
2 eggs
½ tomato, sliced
2 teaspoons olive oil
2 tablespoons feta cheese, low-fat
½ tablespoon rosemary, chopped
Dash of pepper

Directions:
1. Heat oven to 375 degrees Fahrenheit.
2. Open English muffin and toast to your preference.
3. Brush ½ teaspoon olive oil on each open half of the English muffin.
4. Put a skillet with the other teaspoon of olive oil over medium-high heat.
5. Break eggs into skillet and fry to your preference.
6. Plate one half of your English muffin.
7. Place spinach, eggs, tomato, feta cheese, and rosemary on the English muffin in your desired order.
8. Sprinkle pepper over your masterpiece.
9. Close other half of the English muffin overtop and enjoy!

Nutritional Breakdown:
Calories – 411

Fat in grams – 20
Carbs in grams – 32
Fiber in grams – 4
Protein in grams – 26

## Mediterranean Egg-in-the-Hole (makes 2 servings)

Ingredients:
2 slices whole wheat bread
2 eggs
1/3 cup tomatoes, chopped
1 tablespoon feta cheese, crumbled
1 teaspoon olive oil
1 teaspoon fresh oregano, minced

Directions:
1. Using a cup with the opening less than half the size of your bread, press down to make a hole on each bread slice.
2. Place a large non-stick pan with olive oil over stove on medium-high heat.
3. Place bread slices into pan and let sit until lightly toasted. Flip and repeat.
4. Break the eggs into the holes of the bread.
5. Reduce to medium heat and let cook until eggs reach your desired level of done-ness.
6. Remove from heat and plate.
7. Top with tomatoes, feta cheese, and oregano.
8. Enjoy!

Nutritional Breakdown (per one serving):
Calories – 184
Fat in grams – 10
Carbs in grams – 15
Fiber in grams – 3
Protein in grams – 10

## Chicken and Veggie Breakfast Wraps (makes 2 servings)

Ingredients:

2 ounces chicken breast
2 whole wheat tortillas
1 cup kale, steamed and roughly chopped
¼ cup cottage cheese, low-fat
2 eggs
1 egg white
2 ½ tablespoons sweet pepper, chopped
2 tablespoons green onions, chopped
1 tablespoon olive oil
Dash Italian seasoning
Dash pepper

Directions:
1. Rub a large skillet down with ½ tablespoon olive oil.
2. Cook chicken breast to your preference in skillet. Allow to cool, slice into tiny pieces, and then set aside.
3. Rub the skillet again with remaining ½ tablespoon of olive oil.
4. Place skillet over stove on medium heat.
5. Once warm, add sweet pepper and green onions. Stir occasionally until tender, about 2 minutes.
6. Add kale to the skillet and cook for another 2 minutes or until it begins to wilt, stirring occasionally.
7. Mix chicken slices, cottage cheese, eggs, egg white, Italian seasoning, and pepper in a bowl until well-combined.
8. Pour into skillet overtop sweet pepper, onions, and kale.
9. Once mixture sets around edges, lift with a spatula so the uncooked egg goes to the bottom of the pan to cook.
10. Once egg is fully cooked, transfer your masterpiece to a plate or cutting board.
11. Cut in half.
12. Place each half in the center of a tortilla.
13. Fold up the bottom of the tortilla, then fold in both sides.
14. Enjoy!

Nutritional Breakdown (per one serving):

Calories – 310
Fat in grams – 29
Carbs in grams – 26
Fiber in grams – 4
Protein in grams – 20

## LUNCH

### Seafood Pasta (makes 2 servings)

Ingredients:
48 ounces water
114 grams whole wheat spaghetti noodles, uncooked
230 grams shrimp, cleaned
1 cup spinach
2 tablespoons basil, minced
1 ½ tablespoons capers, drained
1 tablespoon lemon juice
1 tablespoon olive oil

Directions:
1. Bring water to a boil and add pasta, cooking by the directions on the box.
2. Halfway through cooking noodles, add shrimp to pot. Let stew until pasta is al dente and shrimp is done, about 3 minutes.
3. Drain the water.
4. Transfer spaghetti, noodles, and shrimp to a bowl.
5. Mix in the basil, capers, lemon juice, and olive oil. Top with spinach.
6. Divide into two separate bowls and enjoy!

Nutritional Breakdown (per one serving):
Calories – 302
Fat in grams – 10
Carbs in grams – 19
Fiber in grams – 3
Protein in grams – 35

### An Elegant Lady's Pizza (makes 2 servings)

Ingredients:

7 ounces whole wheat pizza dough
130 grams artichoke hearts
¾ cup arugula leaves
½ ounce prosciutto, sliced thin
¼ cup low-fat mozzarella, shredded
1 tablespoon Parmesan, shredded
1 tablespoon lemon juice
1 tablespoon pesto
½ tablespoon cornmeal
Cooking spray

Directions:

1. Put oven rack to lowest position.
2. Preheat oven to 500 degrees Fahrenheit.
3. Spray a baking sheet down with cooking spray.
4. Roll dough into an even layer of 7 x 5 inches. Transfer to baking sheet.
5. Smooth the pesto out over the dough, leaving a bit of the outside parameter clean for crust.
6. Scatter shredded mozzarella over pesto.
7. Put pizza with baking sheet on the bottom oven rack. Let bake for 3 minutes or until cheese has melted.
8. Remove pizza from the oven.
9. Chop artichoke into bite-sized chunks. Scatter over mozzarella cheese.
10. Sprinkle sliced prosciutto overtop.
11. Place your masterpiece back into the oven. Let bake for 4 minutes or until crust starts to turn golden-brown.
12. While pizza is baking, toss lemon juice and arugula in a bowl. Remove pizza from oven and immediately top with the lemon juice-arugula mixture.
13. Cut pizza as desired, plate, and enjoy!

Nutrient breakdown (per one serving):

Calories – 330
Fat in grams – 8
Carbs in grams – 50

Fiber in grams – 5
Protein in grams – 16

## Spicy Pita Burgers (makes 4 Pita Burgers)

Ingredients:
230 grams ground chicken
2 whole wheat pitas, cut in half
1 cup lettuce, shredded
¼ cup tomato, coarsely chopped
¼ cup green onions, chopped
¼ cup low-fat plain yoghurt
1 egg white, beaten
2 ½ tablespoons breadcrumbs
1 tablespoon lemon zest
½ tablespoon Italian seasoning
½ tablespoon olive oil
¾ teaspoon oregano, minced
¼ teaspoon pepper

Directions:
1. In a medium-sized bowl, mix together green onions, breadcrumbs, Italian seasoning, pepper, egg white, and ground chicken.
2. Once well-combined, add ½ teaspoon grated lemon rind. Stir until well-incorporated.
3. Transfer mixture to a counter top and divide into 4 portions.
4. Shape the portions into circular patties, about a ¼ inch thick.
5. Put a skillet with the olive oil over medium-high heat.
6. Once skillet is hot, add patties. Cook for about 2 minutes each side or until brown.
7. Once brown, reduce heat to medium and cover. Cook for another 4 minutes.
8. While burgers finish cooking, mix together the remaining lemon rind, yoghurt, and oregano.
9. Remove burgers from heat.

10. Stuff each pita half with evenly divided yoghurt mixture, lettuce, and tomato. Then stuff with burger as well.
11. Plate and enjoy!

Nutrient Breakdown (per one burger):
Calories – 136
Fat in grams – 10
Carbs in grams – 19
Fiber in grams – 2
Protein in grams – 20

## Greek-Style Couscous (makes 3 servings)

Ingredients:
1 cup + 2 ½ tablespoons ounces water
1 cup vegetable broth
210 grams couscous, uncooked
3 ounces marinated artichoke hearts, un-drained
1 ½ cups chicken breast, cooked and diced
½ cup parsley, chopped
¼ cup sun-dried tomatoes
¼ cup feta cheese, crumbled
Dash of pepper

Directions:
1. Put 1 cup water and the sun-dried tomatoes in a microwave safe dish.
2. Microwave for 1 ½ - 2 minutes on high or until water comes to a boil.
3. Remove from microwave, cover, and let sit for 7 minutes or until tomatoes are soft.
4. Drain water from tomatoes and dice. Put aside for later.
5. In a large saucepan, combine vegetable broth with 2 ½ tablespoons water. Bring mixture to a boil.
6. Once mixture has boiled, add the couscous.
7. Stir, cover the saucepan with a lid, and reduce heat to a simmer. Let sit for 6 minutes or until couscous has absorbed liquid and is cooked.

8. Transfer couscous to a bowl and sit in marinated artichoke hearts, chicken breast, parsley, sun-dried tomatoes, feta cheese, and pepper. Once well-combined, divide into three portions.
9. Plate and enjoy with some whole wheat toast or crackers!

Nutrient Breakdown (per one serving):
Calories – 146
Fat in grams – 7
Carbs in grams – 29
Fiber in grams – 3
Protein in grams – 26

## Classic Greek Salad (makes 2 servings)

Ingredients:
1 head romaine lettuce
1 red onion
6 ounces black olives, pit removed
2 sweet peppers of your color preference
2 large tomatoes
1 cucumber
1 cup feta cheese, broken into bite-sized bits
6 tablespoons olive oil
1 teaspoon oregano, dried
1 lemon
Dash of pepper

Directions:
1. Rinse and dry the lettuce, then chop into bite-sized pieces
2. Thinly slice the red onion and cucumber.
3. Dice the sweet peppers and tomatoes.
4. Toss first seven ingredients in a salad bowl.
5. Juice the lemon.
6. Pour olive oil, oregano, lemon juice, and black pepper into a jar. Put the lid on the jar and shake until all ingredients are well incorporated.

7. Pour dressing into the salad bowl.
8. Toss until all veggies are coated in dressing.
9. Portion, serve, and enjoy!

Nutrient Breakdown (per one serving):
Calories – 265
Fat in grams – 22
Carbs in grams – 14
Fiber in grams – 3
Protein in grams – 6

## Mediterranean Pasta Salad (makes 2 servings)

Ingredients:
8 ounces whole wheat penne
½ cup black olives, pitted
2 tablespoons olive oil
½ teaspoon basil
½ teaspoon pepper
½ teaspoon garlic salt
½ teaspoon lemon juice
1 tomato, diced
½ sweet pepper, diced
½ red onion, diced
½ English cucumber, diced

Directions:
1. Cook whole wheat penne to your preference by directions on the box.
2. Once penne is cooked, drain and rinse noodles in cold water.
3. Pour olive oil, basil, pepper, garlic salt, and lemon juice into a jar. Shake until all ingredients are well incorporated.
4. Transfer pasta to a large serving bowl.
5. Add black olives, tomato, sweet pepper, red onion, and cucumber to pasta bowl. Toss until all ingredients are thoroughly combined.
6. Pour dressing from jar over pasta salad.

7. Toss salad until all ingredients have an even coating of dressing.
8. Portion, serve, and enjoy!

Nutrient Breakdown (per one serving):
Calories – 302
Fat in grams – 10
Carbs in grams – 47
Fiber in grams – 0
Protein in grams – 8

## Mediterranean Shish Kebabs (makes 3 kebabs)

Ingredients:
450 grams boneless chicken breast
1 sweet pepper, diced
½ onion, diced
6 mushrooms
6 cherry tomatoes
2 tablespoons lemon juice
2 tablespoons olive oil
2 tablespoons white vinegar
1 clove garlic, finely chopped
½ teaspoon oregano
½ teaspoon cumin
¼ teaspoon thyme
Dash of pepper
wooden skewers

Directions:
1. Pour the lemon juice, olive oil, white vinegar, garlic, oregano, cumin, thyme, and pepper into a jar. Shake until ingredients are well-combined.
2. Cut the boneless chicken breast into bite-sized pieces. Transfer to a glass or ceramic bowl.
3. Pour dressing over chicken breast.
4. Toss chicken breast with dressing until chicken is evenly coated.

5. Place a lid or plastic wrap over the bowl and let sit in the fridge to marinate for 1 hour.
6. Pour a thin layer of water over a plate. Place wooden skewers in water and let soak for 30 minutes.
7. Preheat grill to medium-high heat.
8. Take marinated chicken out of the fridge and remove from bowl, discarding excess marinade.
9. Pierce pieces of chicken, sweet pepper, onion, mushrooms, and cherry tomatoes to create a pattern on the wooden skewers.
10. Grill the skewers, turning occasionally.
11. Take off grill after 10-minutes or once veggies have browned and chicken is fully cooked.
12. Serve with your favorite low-fat dip and enjoy!

Nutrient breakdown (per one skewer):
Calories – 290
Fat in grams – 13
Carbs in grams – 9
Fiber in grams – 2
Protein in grams – 34

**Greek-Approved Fried Rice (makes 2 servings)**

Ingredients:
¾ cup rice, cooked
5 ounces spinach, chopped
3 ounces artichoke hearts, cleaned and diced
2 ounces marinated red peppers, cleaned and diced
¼ cup feta cheese, broken into tiny pieces
1 tablespoon olive oil
½ clove garlic

Directions:
1. Put a pan with the olive oil over medium heat.
2. Once pan is hot, add the garlic. Stir until brown.
3. Add the rice, stirring until it begins to brown as well.
4. Add the spinach. Combine all ingredients evenly and let cook for 3 more minutes.

5. Add the artichoke hearts and roasted red peppers. Stir occasionally for 2 minutes.
6. Sprinkle feta cheese over top and then stir it into your masterpiece until evenly scattered.
7. Transfer onto two plates, serve, and enjoy!

Nutrient Breakdown (per one serving):
Calories – 244
Fat in grams – 13
Carbs in grams – 26
Fiber in grams - 3
Protein in grams – 9

**Spanish Tuna Melts (makes 2 sandwiches)**

Ingredients:
2 slices toast, rye or multigrain
6 ½ ounces oil-packed Tuna, drained with 1 tablespoon oil saved
¼ cup Manchego, grated
¼ cup roasted red pepper, drained and sliced
¼ cup red onion, sliced thin
¼ cup olives, pit removed
1 ½ tablespoons lemon juice
¾ tablespoon almonds, diced
½ tablespoon chives, minced
½ tablespoon olive oil
½ teaspoon lemon rind, grated

Directions:
1. Place oven rack on highest setting.
2. Preheat oven to 400 degrees Fahrenheit.
3. Spread olive oil over bread and place on top rack of oven, about 1-2 minutes each side.
4. Remove bread from oven. Keep oven on.
5. Combine tuna with reserved tuna oil, lemon zest, and lemon juice. While combining, break tuna into bite-sized chunks.

6. Add the roasted red pepper slices, sliced red onion, and pitted olives. Mix until all ingredients are well-combined.
7. Spoon mixture onto baked bread slices, dividing evenly between the two.
8. Sprinkle grated Manchego overtop and place back in the oven until cheese has melted.
9. Top with minced chives and diced almonds.
10. Plate and enjoy!

Nutrient Breakdown (per one tuna melt):
Calories – 421
Fat in grams – 23
Carbs in grams – 28
Fiber in grams – 4
Protein in grams – 29

## Classic Submarine Sandwich (makes 2 sandwiches)

Ingredients:
2 whole wheat sub buns, cut in half lengthwise
115 grams chicken, cooked and sliced
115 grams mozzarella cheese
½ sweet pepper, grilled and diced
2/3 cup mushrooms, grilled and diced
3 tablespoons olive oil
2 tablespoons mayonnaise
2 tablespoons basil leaves, minced
1 tablespoon red wine vinegar

Directions:
1. Preheat oven to 350 degrees Fahrenheit.
2. In a bowl stir together olive oil, mayo, basil, and red wine vinegar until well combined.
3. Spread mixture over the cut face of the buns.
4. Layer buns with chicken, mozzarella, sweet pepper and mushrooms, dividing evenly between the two as you go.
5. Close buns with top half of bread and wrap sandwiches in tin foil.

6. Place in the oven and let sit for about 4 minutes or until mozzarella cheese has melted.
7. Remove from oven and discard tin foil.
8. Plate and enjoy!

Nutrient Breakdown (per 1 sandwich):
Calories – 683
Fat in grams – 43
Carbs in grams – 39
Fiber in grams – 6
Protein in grams – 40

## DINNER

### Salmon with all the Fixings (makes 2 servings)

Ingredients:
2x 6 ounce filet of skinless salmon, 1 inch thick
1 cup cherry tomatoes, cut in half
½ can olives, drained, pitted, and sliced
¼ cup zucchini, diced
1 tablespoon capers
1 ½ tablespoon olive oil
Dash of pepper

Directions:
1. Preheat oven to 425 degrees Fahrenheit.
2. Rub pepper over both sides of salmon.
3. Coat a baking dish with ½ tablespoon olive oil and lay salmon in it.
4. In a medium sized bowl, mix together cherry tomatoes, olives, zucchini, capers, and remaining olive oil.
5. Scatter mixture over top of salmon.
6. Place baking dish in the oven and let bake for 15-20 minutes, or until salmon is cooked through.
7. Plate, serve with some red wine, and enjoy!

Nutrient Breakdown (per one serving):
Calories – 415
Fat in grams – 27

Carbs in grams – 6
Fiber in grams – 3
Protein – 35

## Chickpea Burgers (makes 4 burgers)

Ingredients:
8 ounce can of chickpeas, rinsed and drained
4 cups romaine lettuce, rinsed, dried, and chopped
4 whole wheat burger buns
½ cup cherry tomatoes, cut in half
½ cup whole wheat flour
¼ cup olive oil
¼ cup Greek yoghurt, low-fat
¼ cup red onion, sliced thin
¼ cup parsley, minced
1 small egg, beaten
1 ½ tablespoons lemon juice
1 small garlic clove, minced
¼ teaspoon pepper
Dash cumin

Directions:
1. In a food processor, pulse together chickpeas, parsley, garlic, half the pepper, and cumin until ground up and well-combined.
2. Transfer mixture to a medium-sized bowl.
3. Add a tablespoon of flour and the beaten egg. Fold together with hands until nicely incorporated.
4. Divide mixture and form into burger-shaped patties, about a ½ inch thick.
5. In a small dish, roll burger patties in the remaining flour. Discard excess flour.
6. Place a non-stick skillet with the olive oil over a stove on medium-high heat.
7. Once the oil is hot, add patties. Cook until each side is golden, about 2-3 minutes each side.
8. Spoon Greek yoghurt, lemon juice, and remaining pepper into a jar. Shake until well-combined.

9. Open the burger buns and place a patty down on each bottom half.
10. Top with the greens, drizzle with Greek yoghurt sauce, and close with top half of burger bun.
11. Serve and enjoy!

Nutrient breakdown (per burger):
Calories – 378
Fat in grams – 17
Carbs in grams – 49
Fiber in grams – 6
Protein in grams – 11

**Stuffed Portobello Mushrooms (makes 2 stuffed mushrooms)**

Ingredients:
2x 4-inch Portobello mushroom caps
2 cups salad greens
1 ½ cup French bread, toasted and cubed
¼ cup vegetable broth
¼ cup feta cheese, in crumbs
¼ cup sweet pepper, diced
2 tablespoons onion, minced
2 tablespoons carrot, minced
2 tablespoons celery, minced
1 ½ tablespoon balsamic vinaigrette
1 tablespoon olive oil
1 garlic clove, minced
2 teaspoons Parmesan cheese, grated
Dash of pepper
Dash of Italian seasoning

Directions:
1. Preheat oven to 350 degrees Fahrenheit.
2. Slice stems off of mushrooms.
3. Dice stems to create ¼ cup. Discard the remaining.

4.  In a medium-sized bowl, mix together diced mushroom stems, bell pepper, onion, carrot, celery, garlic, and Italian seasoning until well-combined.
5.  Put a non-stick skillet with half the olive oil over medium heat.
6.  Once pan is hot, add mushroom stem mixture.
7.  Let fry for about 10 minutes or until veggies are soft. Remove from heat.
8.  Transfer mushroom stem mixture back to medium-sized bowl. Add diced French bread and mix until well-combined.
9.  Bit by bit, add vegetable broth to the bowl, tossing as you go.
10. Add feta cheese and toss again.
11. With a spoon, scoop the gills out of the Portobello mushroom caps and discard of them.
12. Rub a baking sheet with the remaining olive oil and place mushrooms on it, stems facing up.
13. Brush mushrooms with ½ tablespoon of balsamic vinaigrette.
14. Top with parmesan, pepper, and mushroom stem mixture (divided evenly over mushrooms).
15. Place baking sheet in the oven and let sit for about 20 minutes or until mushrooms are soft.
16. While the mushrooms are in the oven, toss together remaining balsamic vinaigrette and salad greens.
17. Set the table by spreading dressed salad greens over two plates.
18. Once mushrooms are done, place one on each plate on top of salad greens.
19. Eat with a friend and enjoy!

Nutrient Breakdown (per one serving):
Calories – 182
Fat in grams – 6
Carbs in grams – 23
Fiber in grams – 4
Protein in grams – 9

# Cheesy Eggplant Sandwiches (makes 2 servings)

Ingredients:
1 medium-sized eggplant, diced
2 pieces rustic Italian bread
½ cup sundried tomatoes
½ cup baby spinach
¼ cup low-fat mozzarella cheese, grated
1 ½ tablespoons Parmesan cheese, grated
1 ½ tablespoons basil, minced
1 tablespoon + 1 teaspoon olive oil, divided

Directions:
1. Preheat grill to medium high.
2. Toss diced eggplant with 1 tablespoon olive oil. Place eggplant on a baking sheet.
3. In a small bowl, mix together parmesan and mozzarella.
4. Spread remaining olive oil over both sides of rustic Italian bread.
5. Dump baby spinach into a medium-sized microwave-safe bowl. Cover with a microwave-safe lid that has breathing holes.
6. Put bowl into the microwave for 1 ½ - 2 minutes, or until baby spinach is soft.
7. Dump sundried tomatoes, basil, and 3 tablespoons water into a separate microwave-safe bowl. Stir and cover with a microwave-safe lid that has breathing holes.
8. Place bowl with sundried tomatoes, basil, and water in the microwave for about 1 ½ minutes, or until mixture is bubbling.
9. Top eggplant with microwaved baby spinach, sundried tomatoes, basil, and water. Make sure it is spread evenly across the baking sheet.
10. Place the baking sheet on the grill, pushing ingredients around every so often. Continue to do so until eggplant has browned on both sides.
11. Grill the rustic Italian bread until nicely toasted, about 1 minute each side.

12. Once bread is toasted and eggplant has browned, divide the eggplant mixture and cheeses over the bread slices.
13. With the bread slices on the baking sheet, close the grill lid and let sit about 4-6 minutes or until cheese has melted.
14. Serve with some red wine and enjoy!

Nutrient Breakdown (per one sandwich):
Calories – 480
Fat in grams – 11
Carbs in grams – 75
Fiber in grams – 20
Protein in grams – 25

**Vegetarian Pasta Bolognese (makes 2 servings)**

Ingredients:
7 ounce can of beans, rinsed and drained
7 ounce can of diced tomatoes
4 ounces whole-wheat fettuccine
¼ cup Parmesan cheese, grated
¼ cup carrot, diced
¼ cup white wine
2 tablespoons celery, diced
2 tablespoons parsley
1 tablespoon olive oil
½ small onion, minced
½ bay leaf
2 cloves garlic, minced

Directions:
1. Bring a medium-sized pot to a boil.
2. While water comes to a boil, mash ¼ cup of beans with a potato masher or fork.
3. Place a saucepan with the oil over medium heat.
4. Once oil is hot, add carrot, celery, and onion. Cover with a lid and let cook, stirring occasionally.

5. Once the saucepan veggies are tender, add the garlic and bay leaf and continue to cook about 15 seconds, or until fragrant.
6. Pour the wine into the saucepan. Turn heat up to high and let boil until liquid evaporates.
7. Once liquid has evaporated, add the mashed beans, tomatoes (including juice), and 1 tablespoon parsley.
8. Reduce to a simmer and let sit, stirring occasionally, until the sauce has thickened. This usually takes between 3-5 minutes.
9. Once sauce is thick, stir in the leftover beans.
10. Let sit for about 1 more minute or until whole beans have heated through, stirring occasionally. Remove sauce from heat and discard of the bay leaf.
11. Once the pasta water has come to a boil, add the pasta and cook according to your preferences and the directions on the box. Drain once noodles are cooked.
12. In a large bowl, toss the cooked noodles and sauce until well-combined.
13. Separate into two bowls, sprinkle with parmesan cheese and leftover parsley, and enjoy!

Nutrient Breakdown (per one serving):
Calories – 443
Fat in grams – 11
Carbs in grams – 67
Fiber in grams – 14
Protein in grams – 19

## Spanish Seafood Fried Rice (makes 2 servings)

Ingredients:
8 ounces shrimp, cleaned
8 ounces mussels, cleaned
1 cup instant brown rice
2/3 cup vegetable broth
½ cup peas
¼ cup onion, minced
¼ cup sweet pepper, diced

1 clove garlic, minced
½ tablespoon olive oil
¼ teaspoon dried thyme
Dash of saffron
Dash of pepper

Directions:
1. Put skillet with olive oil over stove on medium heat.
2. Once skillet is hot, add the onion, sweet pepper, and garlic, stirring occasionally.
3. Once veggies have softened, add in the instant brown rice, vegetable broth, thyme, saffron, and pepper. Once mixture comes to a boil cover with a lid and let cook for 3-4 minutes, or until vegetable broth has mostly evaporated.
4. Add in the shrimp and peas, stirring until well-combined.
5. Arrange mussels in an even layer over top of the rice mixture.
6. Cover with the lid again and let steam for another 3-4 minutes, or until the rice is soft and the mussels have opened.
7. Remove from the heat and let stand until the rest of the vegetable broth is absorbed.
8. Divide onto two plates, serve with some red wine, and enjoy!

Nutrient Breakdown (per one serving):
Calories – 371
Fat in grams – 7
Carbs in grams – 44
Fiber in grams – 5
Protein in grams – 30

## Chicken with Greek-Style Quinoa Salad (makes 2 servings)

Ingredients:
200 grams chicken breast

150 grams tomatoes, diced
110 grams quinoa
50 grams feta cheese, crumbled
¼ cup black olives, pits removed
½ red onion, minced
1 small chili pepper, seeds removed and minced
1 tablespoon lemon juice
¾ tablespoon olive oil
3 mint leaves, minced
1 small garlic clove, minced
Sprinkling of lemon zest

Directions:

1. Bring a pot of water to a boil and add the quinoa. Cook according to directions on package.
2. Once quinoa is cooked, rinse with cold water and drain. Place in the fridge.
3. In a small bowl, mix together ¾ of the olive oil, chili, and garlic until well-combined.
4. Drizzle remaining olive oil into a medium-sized bowl. Add chicken and toss until chicken has an even coating.
5. Place a pan over a stove on medium-high heat.
6. Once the pan is hot, add the olive-oil coated chicken. Cook for about 3-4 minutes each side or until middle is no longer pink.
7. Set cooked chicken on a plate. Evenly distribute the chili-garlic sauce over chicken and allow it to melt. Set aside.
8. In a medium sized bowl, toss together tomatoes, black olives, red onion, feta cheese, and mint. Add the quinoa and toss again.
9. Once quinoa and veggies are evenly distributed, dump in the lemon juice and zest. Toss again until well-incorporated.
10. Portion the quinoa salad on two plates and top with the seasoned chicken breast.
11. Serve with some red wine and enjoy!

Nutrient Breakdown (per one serving):

Calories – 431
Fat in grams – 21
Carbs in grams – 24
Fiber in grams – 3
Protein in grams – 25

## Italian Potato Salad (makes 2 servings)

Ingredients:
7 ounces cherry tomatoes
5 ounces potatoes, cut into bite-sized chunks
2 ounces roasted red peppers from a jar, chopped
½ ounce black olives, chopped
½ tablespoon olive oil
½ teaspoon oregano
½ small onion, minced
3 basil leaves, minced
1 small garlic clove, minced

Directions:
1. Start to boil a large pot of water for the potatoes.
2. Put a saucepan with the olive oil over medium heat.
3. Once the oil is hot, add the onion and cook until tender, about 4-7 minutes.
4. Mix in the oregano and garlic. Let cook for another minute.
5. Mix in the cherry tomatoes and roasted red peppers. Reduce heat to a simmer and let sit for 7 minutes.
6. While ingredients in the saucepan simmer, add the potatoes to the large pot of boiling water. Let cook until soft, about 9-12 minutes.
7. Once potatoes are cooked through, drain the water.
8. Transfer potatoes to large bowl and drizzle saucepan mixture over top. Gently toss until all the potatoes are coated in sauce.
9. Portion into 2 servings and enjoy!

Nutrient Breakdown (per one serving):
Calories – 111

Fat in grams – 4
Carbs in grams – 16
Fiber in grams – 2
Protein in grams – 3

## Roasted Veggies (makes 2 servings)

Ingredients:
225 grams butternut squash, peeled and diced into bite-sized pieces
100 grams polenta
100 grams raw beetroot, diced into bite-sized pieces
60 grams arugula
30 grams parmesan cheese, grated
½ medium red onion, sliced into wedges
3 tablespoons olive oil
1 tablespoon lemon juice
1 teaspoon thyme leaves
Dash of pepper

Directions:
1. Preheat oven to 390 degrees Fahrenheit.
2. In a small bowl, toss together the parmesan cheese and pepper. Sprinkle the mixture over a baking sheet covered in parchment paper.
3. Place the baking sheet in the oven for 3 minutes, or until cheese begins to turn golden.
4. Remove baking sheet from oven and allow to cool for 5 minutes. Then, crush the melted parmesan into bite-sized pieces.
5. Turn the oven up to 430 degrees Fahrenheit.
6. In a medium-sized bowl, toss together squash, beetroot, lemon juice, pepper, and half the olive oil until thoroughly distributed.
7. Transfer mixture from bowl to a roasting pan. Place roasting pan in the oven for 15 minutes.
8. Add onion wedges to roasting tin at 15 minutes. Bake for another 3 minutes.

9. While squash and beetroot are in the oven, bring ½ a litre of water to a boil.
10. While water comes to a bowl, put a large pot with half of the remaining olive oil over medium-low heat.
11. Once olive oil is hot, dump in the polenta and let simmer until cooked according to the directions on the box. TIP: If polenta is too dry, stir in ½ cup of water.
12. Once polenta reaches your desired consistency, stir in the remaining oil and baked parmesan pieces until well-combined.
13. Portion the polenta on to two plates and top with baked squash and beetroot. Top with arugula and thyme.
14. Serve with a glass of red wine and enjoy!

Nutrient Breakdown (per one serving):
Calories – 375
Fat in grams – 25
Carbs in grams – 61
Fiber in grams – 9
Protein in grams – 10

## Breadcrumbs for Dinner (makes 2 servings)

Ingredients:
18 ounces spinach
3 ½ ounces whole wheat bread crumbs
1 ½ tablespoons olive oil
2 garlic cloves, minced
1 chili, minced
Zest of 1 lemon

Directions:
1. Place a large frying pan with the olive oil over medium heat.
2. Once the oil is hot, add the whole wheat bread crumbs, garlic, chili, and lemon zest. Let sit until breadcrumbs are slightly browned and crispy.
3. Transfer mixture into a bowl and set aside.

4. To the same pan, add the spinach. Keep stirring until it begins to wilt.
5. Portion on two plates and top with breadcrumb mixture.
6. Serve and enjoy!

Nutrient Breakdown (per one serving):
Calories – 368
Fat in grams – 14
Carbs in grams – 51
Fiber in grams – 11
Protein in grams – 13

# SNACKS

## Feta Cheese and Olives Marinade (makes 2 cups)

Ingredients:
1 1/3 cup black olives, pitted and sliced
½ cup low-fat feta cheese, diced
2 ½ tablespoons olive oil
2 cloves garlic, minced
Juice of 1 lemon
Zest of 1 lemon
1 heaping teaspoon rosemary, minced
Dash of cayenne pepper
Dash of pepper

Directions:
1. In a medium-sized bowl, mix together olives, feta cheese, olive oil, garlic, lemon juice, lemon zest, rosemary, cayenne pepper, and pepper.
2. Cover the bowl with plastic wrap and place in the fridge for a few hours to let flavors pull through.
3. Serve over some whole wheat toast to share with family and friends!

Nutrient Breakdown (per 1 tablespoon):
Calories – 37
Fat in grams – 4

Carbs in grams – 1
Fiber in grams – 0
Protein in grams – 1

## Tomato Tea Party Sandwiches (makes 2 sandwiches)

Ingredients:
2 whole wheat bread slices
4 teaspoons olive oil
2 teaspoons basil, minced
2 thick tomato slices
Dash of pepper

Directions:
1. Toast bread to your desired level of doneness.
2. Spread 2 teaspoons olive oil on each slice of bread.
3. Top with tomato, then sprinkle with basil and pepper.
4. Serve with lemon water and enjoy!

Nutrient Breakdown (per one sandwich):
Calories – 75
Fat in grams – 2
Carbs in grams – 12
Fiber in grams – 2
Protein in grams – 2

## Dates in a Blanket (makes 8 pieces)

Ingredients:
2 pieces prosciutto, sliced lengthwise into 4 pieces each
8 fresh dates
Dash of pepper

Directions:
1. Wrap each date with a slice of prosciutto.
1. Sprinkle with pepper.
2. Serve and enjoy!

Nutrient Breakdown (per one piece):
Calories – 39

Fat in grams – 1
Carbs in grams – 6
Fiber in grams – 1
Protein in grams – 2

## Veggie Shish Kebabs (makes 8 pieces)

Ingredients:
8 wooden skewers
8 cherry tomatoes
8 low-fat mozzarella balls
8 basil leaves
1 teaspoon olive oil
Dash of pepper

Directions:
1. Stab 1 cherry tomato, low-fat mozzarella ball, and basil leaf onto each skewer.
2. Place skewers on a plate and drizzle with olive oil. Finish with a sprinkle of pepper.
3. Enjoy!

Nutrient Breakdown (per one skewer):
Calories – 46
Fat in grams – 3
Carbs in grams – 1
Fiber in grams – 0
Protein in grams – 3

## Mediterranean Sushi (makes 6 rolls)

Ingredients:
1 large English cucumber
3 tablespoons sun-dried tomatoes, diced
3 tablespoons hummus
3 tablespoons low-fat feta cheese, crumbled
2 cloves garlic, minced
Dash pepper

Directions:

1. Using a vegetable sheer, peel the outside skin off the cucumber.
2. Once cucumber is peeled, create 6 thin pieces by slicing lengthwise.
3. Lay cucumber slices out side-by-side on a cutting board.
4. Layer about 1 ½ teaspoons of hummus over each cucumber slice.
5. Top each slice with 1 ½ teaspoons sun-dried tomatoes and low-fat feta cheese.
6. Sprinkle with pepper.
7. Pick up the end of a cucumber slice that's closest to you and begin to roll so that ingredients are on the inside. TIP: Don't roll too tight or the filling will squish out.
8. Secure each roll with a toothpick.
9. Repeat steps 8-9 for the remaining slices of cucumber.
10. Plate and enjoy!

Nutrient Breakdown (per one roll):
Calories – 35
Fat in grams – 1
Carbs in grams – 5
Fiber in grams – 1
Protein in grams – 8

**Roasted Chickpeas (makes 1 serving or 1 cup)**

Ingredients:
15 ounce can of chickpeas
1 clove garlic, minced
1 tablespoon olive oil
1 teaspoon lemon juice
1 teaspoon red wine vinegar
¼ teaspoon garlic powder
¼ teaspoon pepper

Directions:
1. Preheat oven to 425 degrees Fahrenheit.
2. Line a baking sheet with parchment paper.

3. Drain and rinse the chickpeas. Dry with a paper towel.
4. Spread chickpeas over parchment paper in an even layer.
5. Place the baking sheet into the oven and roast for 5-7 minutes.
6. Turn the chickpeas over with a spatula. Then roast for another 5-7 minutes.
7. While the chickpeas finish roasting, stir together garlic, olive oil, lemon juice, red wine vinegar, garlic powder, and pepper in a medium-sized bowl.
8. Take the chickpeas out of the oven and add them to the mixture in the large bowl. Toss until chickpeas have an even coating of the mixture.
9. Transfer the chickpeas back onto the roasting pan and place back into the oven for another 4-7 minutes, or until they are crispy.
10. Remove from the oven, let them cool, and enjoy!

Nutrient Breakdown:
Calories – 167
Fat in grams – 20
Carbs in grams – 62
Fiber in grams – 20
Protein in grams – 20

**Sweet-Baked Banana (makes two servings)**

Ingredients:
2 ripe bananas
4 teaspoons honey
1 ½ teaspoons cinnamon

Directions:
1. Preheat oven to 350 degrees Fahrenheit.
2. Slice bananas into bite sized chunks.
3. Pour honey and cinnamon until a medium-sized bowl. Mix until cinnamon is evenly spread through honey.
4. Add bananas and gently toss until they have an even coating.

5. Transfer bananas onto a lined baking sheet. Spread them into one even layer.
6. Place baking sheet into the oven and bake for 10-15 minutes or until bananas are slightly browned.
7. Portion into 2 bowls and enjoy!

Nutrient Breakdown (per one serving):
Calories – 151
Fat in grams – 0
Carbs in grams – 40
Fiber in grams – 4
Protein in grams – 1

## Spicy Red Pepper Spread (makes 2 cups)

Ingredients:
4 red sweet peppers, seeded, skinned, and roasted
2 guajillo chilies, dried
½ cup pumpkin seeds, shelled and toasted
1/3 cup olive oil
2 tablespoons tomato paste
1 1/3 teaspoon red wine vinegar
1 teaspoon paprika
2 garlic cloves, minced
Dash of pepper

Directions:
1. Bring 2 cups of water to a boil.
2. Pour boiling water into a medium-sized bowl, over the guajillo chilies.
3. Press guajillo chilies to the bottom of the bowl by setting a spoon or glass over them. Let soak for 40 minutes.
4. Drain water from bowl.
5. Remove the guajillo chilies stem and seeds, then dice.
6. Transfer the diced guajillo chilies into a food processor. Add the red sweet peppers, pumpkin seeds, olive oil, tomato paste, red wine vinegar, and paprika and pulse until mixture comes to a smooth paste.

7. Transfer to a serving dish and stir in the pepper.
8. Leave dip to sit in room temperature for 40 minutes so that the flavors pull through.
9. Serve with some veggies and enjoy!

Nutrient Breakdown (per ¼ cup):
Calories – 157
Fat in grams – 13
Carbs in grams – 11
Fiber in grams – 2
Protein in grams – 4

## Tomato Poached Mozzarella Balls (makes 4 balls)

Ingredients:
8 medium tomatoes, peeled, seeded, and diced
4 small mozzarella cheese balls, drained
2 ½ tablespoons basil leaves plus extra to garnish
2 ½ tablespoons olive oil
3 small garlic cloves, minced
Dash of pepper

Directions:
1. Put a large saucepan with the olive oil over medium heat.
2. Once the oil is hot, dump in the minced garlic and fry, stirring occasionally, until garlic is slightly browned.
3. Strain the garlic from the oil and discard of it.
4. Turn the stove down to medium-low heat.
5. Dump in the diced tomatoes and let simmer until tomatoes are mostly liquid.
6. Season with pepper and let cool.
7. Once tomatoes have cooled, transfer them to a blender. Pulse until a smooth paste is created.
8. Transfer the tomato mixture back into the large saucepan and bring to a simmer.
9. Place the mozzarella balls in the simmering tomato mixture and remove from the heat. Let sit for 5-7 minutes.

10. While the mozzarella balls bathe in the tomato mixture, mince the basil.
11. Remove the mozzarella balls from the tomato mixture and place each on a plate.
12. Stir the minced basil in the sauce until nicely incorporated.
13. Portion sauce onto each mozzarella ball and top with extra basil.
14. Enjoy on its own or with a piece of whole wheat bread!

Nutrient Breakdown (per one ball):
Calories – 176
Fat in grams – 13
Carbs in grams – 11
Fiber in grams – 3
Protein in grams – 7

## Mini Shrimp Cakes (makes 12 pieces)

Ingredients:
24 small shrimps, cleaned
12 cilantro leaves
2-3 radishes, cleaned and sliced into 12 rounds
1-2 hearts of palm, cleaned and sliced into 12 rounds
1 tablespoon of lime juice
1 tablespoon olive oil
½ tablespoon mayonnaise
Dash of coriander
Dash of lime zest
Dash of cayenne
Dash of pepper

Directions:
1. Lay the palm rounds out on a serving platter.
2. Pour over the lime juice, olive oil, and 1 ½ tablespoons water.
3. Gently shake the dish to evenly distribute toppings.
4. Stir together mayonnaise, coriander, lime zest, cayenne, and pepper in a small-sized bowl.

5. Add the shrimp and toss until evenly coated.
6. With a paper towel, absorb the liquid seasonings off of the palm rounds.
7. Place a radish round atop each palm round.
8. Top each round tower with two mayonnaise coated shrimp and a cilantro leaf.
9. Serve and enjoy!

Nutrient Breakdown (per one piece):
Calories – 30
Fat in grams – 2
Carbs in grams – 1
Fiber in grams – 0
Protein in grams – 2


## DESSERT

### Grilled Peaches and Cream (makes 2 servings)

Peaches Ingredients:
2 peaches
1/2 cup low-fat sugar-free whipped cream
1/4 cup blueberries
1/2 tablespoon dukkah
1 teaspoon olive oil

Dukkah Ingredients:
2 1/2 tablespoons almonds, toasted
2 1/2 pistachios, toasted
1/2 tablespoon caraway seeds
1/2 tablespoon coriander seeds
1/2 tablespoons cumin seeds

Other Topping Ingredients:
1 1/2 tablespoons sesame seeds, toasted
1/2 teaspoon Aleppo pepper
1/2 teaspoon mint
1/2 teaspoon lemon zest
1/4 teaspoon dried marjoram

Dukkah Directions:
1. Dice the almonds and pistachios.
2. Using an electric coffee grinder, mince the caraway, coriander, and cumin seeds.
3. Transfer the ground caraway, coriander, and cumin into a bowl. Stir in sesame seeds, Aleppo pepper, mint, lemon zest, and dried marjoram until well combined.
4. Scoop into a jar and seal tightly. Set aside.

Peaches Directions:
1. Turn on grill.
2. While grill heats up, halve the peaches and remove the pits.
3. Brush peaches with olive oil.
4. Place peaches on the grill cut-side down and let grill for 5 minutes. TIP: Do not turn the peaches.
5. Portion peaches on to two plates.
6. Spread Dukkah over peaches. Top with whipped cream and blueberries.
7. Serve and enjoy!

Nutrient Breakdown (per one serving):
Calories – 140
Fat in grams – 6
Carbs in grams – 21
Fiber in grams – 2
Protein in grams – 2

**Toasted Sesame Ganache (makes 20 chocolates)**

Ingredients:
6 1/4 ounces dark chocolate, 66% or more
1/3 cup sesame seeds
2 1/2 tablespoon tahini
1 1/4 tablespoon honey

Directions:
1. Break the chocolate into pieces and place in a medium-sized bowl. Set aside.

2. Put a saucepan with the honey and a 1/3 cup of water over medium-low heat. Reduce once brought to a simmer.
3. Stir in the tahini and let simmer for 1 minute.
4. Pour hot mixture into the bowl with the chocolate. Whisk ingredients until chocolate has melted and mixture is smooth.
5. Place bowl in the fridge and let sit for about 1 1/2 hours or until hard.
6. While the ganache sets, use a dry frying pan over low heat to lightly toast the sesame seeds. TIP: They are done when they've turned golden but have not yet popped open.
7. Allow cool until ganache in ready.
8. Remove ganache from refrigerator and divide into 20 chocolates with a teaspoon.
9. Roll each chocolate in sesame seeds and eat sparingly!

Nutrient Breakdown (per one chocolate):
Calories – 77
Fat in grams – 5
Carbs in grams – 6
Fiber in grams – 1
Protein in grams – 1

**Warm, sweet, hot cherries (makes 5 cups)**

Ingredients:
2 lb cherries, pits removed
3 1/2 cups water
6 strips lemon zest
6 strips orange zest
1/2 vanilla bean, split open
30 peppercorns

Directions:
1. Put a large saucepan with the water, lemon zest, orange zest, vanilla bean, and peppercorn over high heat. Reduce to medium-low once it comes to a boil.

2. Dump in the cherries and simmer for about 7 minutes, or until they are tender without falling apart. TIP: Scoop away foam as you go.
3. Transfer mixture into a large bowl and let sit in the fridge for about an hour, or until cool.
4. Remove from the fridge, discard of vanilla bean, and drain away liquid.
5. Serve with some low-fat sugar-free whipped cream or over low-fat naturally-sweetened gelato and enjoy!

Nutrient Breakdown (per 1 cup):
Calories – 113
Fats in grams – 0
Carbs in grams – 30
Fiber in grams – 4
Protein in grams – 2

**Walnut Spice Bars (makes 15 bars)**

Ingredients:
9 ounces whole wheat frozen puff pastry
1/3 cup + 2 tablespoons honey
1 cup walnuts, chopped
3 tablespoons olive oil
1 1/2 teaspoon cinnamon
1 teaspoon ground ginger
1 egg

Directions:
1. Heat oven to 400 degrees Fahrenheit.
2. Pour the honey, olive oil, cinnamon, and ginger into a food processor. Pulse until all ingredients are well-incorporated and mixture is smooth.
3. Crack the egg into the food processor and pulse again until well-incorporated.
4. Dump the nuts into the food processor and pulse again until well-incorporated. TIP: Nuts shouldn't become so fine that the mixture becomes a paste. The bars taste great with some crunch.

5. Cut the pastry into 22 x 10 centimeter strips. Roll until they become 38 x 15 centimeter strips.
6. Prick the entire length of the strips with a fork.
7. Place strips on a lined baking sheet. Spread nut mixture over each strip, leaving 1 1/2 centimeter of the lengthwise edges bare.
8. Fold the bare edges 1 inch inwards and press into the nut mixture so they stick. Using a table knife, create indentations in these edges about a 1 centimeter apart. This should create a pretty, crimped crust for your bars.
9. Place the baking sheet in the oven and bake for 18-20 minutes, or until filling looks a little bit dry and pastry is a golden-brown.
10. Cut into 3 strips lengthwise and 5 strips widthwise.
11. Serve and enjoy!

Nutrient Breakdown (per one bar):
Calories – 199
Fat in grams – 14
Carbs in grams – 17
Fiber in grams – 1
Protein in grams – 3

## Nutty Banana Bread (makes 1 loaf)

Ingredients:
3 brown bananas
¾ cup almond flour
¾ cup tapioca starch
½ cup walnuts, chopped
½ cup coconut oil
½ cup coconut sugar
1/3 cup canned coconut milk
2 eggs
1 tablespoon lemon juice
1 teaspoon Stevia (powder form)
¾ teaspoons baking powder
½ teaspoon baking soda

Directions:

1. Preheat oven to 350 degrees Fahrenheit.
2. Rub a bread loaf pan with the olive oil.
3. In a large bowl, mix together the bananas, coconut oil, coconut milk, eggs, and lemon juice with an electric hand mixer.
4. In another medium-sized bowl, whisk together almond flour, tapioca starch, coconut sugar, walnuts, Stevia, baking powder, and baking soda.
5. Pour the dry ingredients into the large bowl with the wet ingredients.
6. Mix with the electric hand mixer until all ingredients are well-combined.
7. Transfer the batter into the greased bread loaf pan.
8. Place the pan into the oven and let bake for 30-40 minutes or until fork comes out clean.
9. Cool, slice into 8 pieces, and enjoy!

Nutrient Breakdown (per piece):
Calories – 330
Fat in grams – 25
Carbs in grams – 25
Fiber in grams – 3
Protein in grams – 5

**Greek Almond Cake (makes 10 servings)**

Cake Ingredients:
5 eggs
8 ounces low-fat Greek Yoghurt
8 ounces fruit sugar
7 ounces semolina
5 1/3 ounces whole-wheat flour
2 ½ ounces almonds, ground
¾ cup olive oil
The zest of 1 lemon
The juice of 1 lemon

Icing Ingredients:

1 ½ cups pistachios, shells removed
1 cup honey
The juice of 2 lemons
The zest of 1 lemon
The juice of one orange
The zest of one orange

Directions:
1. Preheat oven to 180 degrees Fahrenheit.
2. In a large bowl, mix the eggs, low-fat Greek yoghurt, fruit sugar, semolina, whole-wheat flour, ground almonds, olive oil, lemon zest, and lemon juice.
3. Rub a 9 inch cake pan with olive oil and sprinkle with a light coating of flour.
4. Pour cake batter into the cake pan.
5. Place cake pan in the oven and bake for 35-40 minutes.
6. Pour the honey, lemon juice, lemon zest, orange juice, and orange zest into a saucepan over medium-low heat. Let it come to a simmer and then let it simmer for 11-15 minutes. The icing should be thick and syrup-like at this point.
7. Take icing off heat and stir in the pistachios. Set aside.
8. Remove cake pan from the oven and let cool until firm.
9. Transfer cake onto a large plate and let cool completely.
10. Once cake is cool, use a wooden skewer to poke holes in the cake.
11. Pour the icing over the cake and let syrup sink into holes.
12. Slice into 10 pieces and enjoy!

Nutrient Breakdown (per one serving):
Calories – 522
Fat in grams – 31
Carbs in grams – 52
Fiber in grams – 5
Protein in grams – 14

**Pistachio Batter Cake (makes 10 servings)**

Cake Ingredients:
4 tablespoons whole-wheat flour
3 ¾ tablespoons fruit sugar
2 ½ tablespoons pistachios
2 ½ tablespoons blanched almonds
4 egg whites
2 egg yolks
1 egg
½ teaspoon cream of tartar
Dash of Stevia (powder form)

Icing Ingredients:
225 grams mascarpone cheese
1 cup heavy cream
Dash of Stevia (powder form)

Directions:
1. Preheat oven to 425 degrees Fahrenheit.
2. In a food processor, pulse pistachios, blanched almonds, and Stevia until nuts are nicely ground.
3. Transfer pulsed nuts and Stevia into a large mixing bowl.
4. Beat in the eggs and egg yolks until thoroughly incorporated.
5. Beat in the egg whites, cream of tartar, and 3 1/3 tablespoons fruit sugar until stiff white peaks form. TIP: It's important to add the fruit sugar a little bit at a time.
6. Pour whole-wheat flour in a little at a time, stirring to fold in as you go.
7. Rub two rectangular cake pans with olive oil.
8. Pour the batter into the pans, dividing evenly.
9. Place cake pans in the oven and let bake for 6-8 minutes, or until a fork comes out clean.
10. Remove the cake pans from the oven and let cool.
11. Remove the cakes from their pans by running a knife or spatula around the edges to loosen.
12. Let cool completely.

13. While cake cools, boil the remaining fruit sugar and ½ cup water in a saucepan until sugar dissolves. Remove from heat and allow to cool.
14. In a medium-sized bowl, beat together mascarpone cheese, heavy cream, and Stevia with an electric hand mixer until well-combined. TIP: You will know ingredients are well-combined once white peaks begin to form.
15. Once cake has completely cooled, spread the sugar syrup over them.
16. Spread frosting over one cake and top with the other cake. Then, spread frosting over this cake as well.
17. Let frosting set in the fridge and cut into 10 pieces.
18. Plate, serve, and enjoy!

Nutrient Breakdown (per one serving):
Calories – 246
Fat in grams – 24
Carbs in grams – 8
Fiber in grams – 1
Protein in grams – 6

## Chia Chocolate Balls (makes 28 balls)

Ingredients:
1 ½ cups oats
¾ cup seed butter
2/3 cup ground flaxseed
½ cup agave
½ cup shredded coconut, unsweetened
¼ cup almonds, chopped
2 tablespoons chia seeds
2 tablespoons cocoa powder
2 teaspoons vanilla extract
½ teaspoon ground cinnamon

Directions:

1. In a large bowl, mix together oats, ground flaxseed, shredded coconut, chopped almonds, chia seeds, cocoa powder, and cinnamon.
2. In a separate bowl, mix together seed butter, agave, and vanilla extract.
3. Bit by bit, beat the dry ingredients until the wet ingredients until well combined.
4. Place mixture in the fridge for about an hour or until nicely chilled.
5. Create 28 rounded balls with the mixture.
6. Enjoy for days to come! TIP: Store in a tightly sealed container in the fridge.

Nutrient Breakdown (per one ball):
Calories – 110
Fat in grams – 7
Carbs in grams – 10
Fiber in grams – 3
Protein in grams – 3

## Simple Gelato (makes 4 servings)

TIP: Eat this one sparingly or only on a day you've done really well for yourself! It does contain sugar which the Mediterranean diet tried to eliminate to your diet. You can store it in your freezer for weeks, no problem!

Ingredients:
3 cups low fat sour cream
2 cups sweetened condensed milk
2 teaspoons vanilla extract

Directions:
1. Whisk all ingredients together in a large bowl until all sour cream lumps disappear. You want it to be smooth and creamy!
2. Transfer the mixture into an air-tight container and freeze overnight.
3. Serve with fresh fruit to top and enjoy!

Nutrient Breakdown (per one serving):
Calories – 408
Fat in grams – 6
Carbs in grams – 74
Fiber in grams – 0
Protein in grams – 12

## Peanut Butter Chocolate Chip Cookies (makes 24 cookies)

Ingredients:
1 2/3 cup quick oats
½ cup dark chocolate chips
½ cup natural peanut butter
1/3 cup coconut palm sugar
¼ cup honey
1 ½ tablespoons olive oil
¾ tablespoon baking soda
½ teaspoon chia seeds
1 egg

Directions:
1. Preheat oven to 350 degrees Fahrenheit.
2. Beat the coconut palm sugar, honey, and olive oil in a medium-sized bowl until smooth.
3. Beat in the natural peanut butter, baking soda, chia seed, and egg until well-combined.
4. Bit by bit, beat in the oats until thoroughly incorporated.
5. Using a wooden spoon, stir in the dark chocolate chips.
6. Line a baking sheet with parchment paper.
7. Portion the mixture into 24 cookies and line the baking sheet with them.
8. Place the baking sheet in the oven and let bake for 5-7 minutes or until cookies start to brown around the edges.
9. Remove the baking pan from the oven and let the cookies cool.
10. Store in an air-tight container and enjoy!

Nutrient Breakdown (per one cookie):
Calories – 110
Fat in grams – 5
Carbs in grams – 18
Fiber in grams – 1
Protein in grams – 2

# Chapter 6 – 7 Days of Food

I created this 7 day meal plan with the intention of helping you get started or helping you get out of a cooking rut, should you ever get stuck in one. Included you will find some recipes as seen in the 50 Scrumptious Recipes chapter that have been shortened for your convenience, plus some simple snacks you can throw together on the fly. At the bottom, you will see a total Nutrient Breakdown so you can accurately determine your daily calorie counts. You will find that some days are better tailored to your needs than others, but don't fret! There are alteration suggestions included in the next chapter to ensure you get your proper fill every day of the week. Bon appetite!

## <u>Sunday</u>

### Breakfast

Fluffy Mediterranean Pancakes
TL;DR In a bowl, whisk together ¾ cup low-fat yoghurt, 1/3 cup fat free milk, and 1 small egg until bubbly. Stir in ½ cup whole wheat pancake mix. Make 10 pancakes, frying 2-3 minutes each side. Top with ½ cup strawberries and 1 tbsp maple syrup. Eat 5 now and save 5 for Tuesday.

### Mid-morning Snack

½ sliced cucumber with ¼ cup Spicy Red Pepper Spread to dip.
TL;DR Let 2 cleaned guajillo chilies soak in boiling water for 40 minutes. Pulse chilies, red sweet peppers, pumpkin seeds, olive oil, tomato paste, red wine vinegar, paprika, and a dash of pepper in a food processor until smooth. Let sit for 40 minutes before eating.

### Lunch

Seafood Pasta
TL;DR Boil 114g whole wheat spaghetti in 48 ounces water. Add 230g shrimp once noodles are half done. Drain and mix with 2 tbsp minced basil, 1 ½ tbsp. drained capers, 1 tbsp lemon juice, and 1 tbsp olive oil. Top with 1 cup spinach and save half for Tuesday's lunch.

## Afternoon Snack

Five walnuts and an orange.

## Dinner

Italian Potato Salad
TL;DR Fry ½ small minced onion, ½ tsp oregano, and 1 clove minced garlic in ½ tbsp. olive oil over medium heat until tender. Add 7 oz cherry tomatoes and 2 oz chopped roasted red peppers, letting simmer for 7 minutes. Cook 5 oz diced potatoes in boiling water and toss in cherry tomato mixture. Eat ½ today and save the other half for Tuesday's dinner.

## Nutrient Breakdown

Calories – 1505
Fat in grams – 60
Carbs in grams – 151
Fiber in grams –17
Protein in grams – 76

# Monday

## Breakfast

Green Eggs and Toast
TL;DR Mash an avocado with 1 tbsp minced mint, ½ tablespoon lemon juice, and a dash of pepper. Spread onto 2 pieces of whole-wheat toast and top with an egg. Sprinkle with 1 ½ ounces feta cheese and pepper.

## Mid-morning Snack

Dates in a blanket
TL;DR Slice a piece of prosciutto into 4 lengthwise pieces. Wrap a fresh date in each piece of prosciutto. Sprinkle with pepper.

## Lunch

Greek-Style Couscous
TL;DR Microwave 1 cup water and ¼ cup sun-dried tomatoes for 2 minutes. Let sit for 7 and drain water. Cook 210 grams couscous in 1 cup vegetable broth and 2 ½ tbsp water. Mix cooked couscous with 3 oz marinated artichoke hearts, 1 ½ cups cooked and diced chicken breast, ½ cup chopped parsley, sun-dried tomatoes, ¼ cup crumbled feta cheese, and a dash of pepper. Make 3 portions – saving 1 for Wednesday and Friday's lunch.

## Afternoon Snack

10 almonds and 10 grapes (frozen grapes are awesome).

## Dinner

Cheesy Eggplant Sandwich
TL;DR
Microwave ½ cup baby spinach until soft. Microwave sundried tomatoes, basil, and 1 ½ tbsp water until bubbling. Mix microwaved contents with ½ diced eggplant and ½ tbsp olive oil. Grill on medium-high until eggplant is slightly browned. Spread ½ tsp. olive oil over a piece of rustic Italian bread and grill. Top with grilled eggplant mixture, 2 tbsp. grated low-fat mozzarella, and ¾ tbsp. grated parmesan. Close grill lid over sandwich until cheese has melted.

## Nutrient Breakdown

Calories – 1486
Fat in grams – 80
Carbs in grams – 198

Fiber in grams – 52
Protein in grams – 95

# Tuesday

### Breakfast

Five Fluffy Mediterranean Pancakes leftover from Monday's breakfast.

### Mid-morning Snack

Five walnuts and an orange.

### Lunch

Reheat leftover Seafood Pasta from Sunday's lunch.

### Afternoon Snack

Two stalks celery with ¼ cup Spicy Red Pepper Spread to dip.

### Dinner

Remaining ½ of the Italian Potato Salad from Sunday's dinner.

### Nutrient Breakdown

Calories – 1509
Fat in grams – 60
Carbs in grams – 151
Fiber in grams – 17
Protein in grams – 76

# Wednesday

### Breakfast

Good Morning Couscous

TL;DR Cook 1 ½ cups milk and an inch of a cinnamon stick over medium-high until bubbles form around edges. Take off heat and stir in ½ cup whole-grain couscous, 2 tbsp dried currants, and 2 tsp brown sugar. Cover and let sit for 15 minutes. Remove cinnamon stick and top with 1 tsp brown sugar. Eat half now and save half for Friday.

## Mid-morning Snack

Baguette topped with Feta Cheese and Olives Marinade
TL;DR Mix together 1 1/3 cup black olives, ½ cup low-fat feta, 2 ½ tbsp olive oil, 2 cloves minced garlic, juice of 1 lemon, zest of 1 lemon, 1 tsp minced rosemary, a dash of cayenne pepper, and a dash of pepper. Cover and refrigerate for a few hours before serving on 4 thin French baguette slices. Eat half today and save half for Friday's afternoon snack.

## Lunch

One portion of the Greek-Style Couscous from Tuesday's lunch.

## Afternoon Snack

½ cup plain low-fat Greek yoghurt topped with ½ cup blackberries and 1 tsp honey.

## Dinner

Vegetarian Pasta Bolognese
TL;DR Fry 1 tbsp olive oil, ¼ cup diced carrot, 2 tbsp diced celery, and ½ small minced onion covered on medium heat. Once tender, add 2 cloves minced garlic, ½ bay leaf, and 2 tbsp white wine. Once wine evaporates, add ¼ cup mashed beans, tomatoes, and 1 tbsp parsley. Allow simmering until sauce is thick and then stir in 5 oz beans. Cook 4 ounces whole wheat pasta and drain. Combine pasta with sauce and sprinkle with ¼ cup grated parmesan cheese and 1 tbsp parsley. Eat ½ today, and save ½ for Friday's dinner.

## Nutrient Breakdown

Calories – 1756
Fat in grams – 90
Carbs in grams – 220
Fiber in grams – 29
Protein in grams – 83

# Thursday

### Breakfast

Fruity Yoghurt Parfait
TL;DR Bit by bit, scoop alternate layers of 6 oz low-fat yoghurt, 1 cup raspberries, and 2 tablespoons granola into a tall glass.

### Mid-morning Snack

Ten baby carrots with ¼ cup Spicy Red Pepper Spread to dip.

### Lunch

Classic Greek Salad
TL;DR Toss a salad of 1 head romaine, 1 red onion, 6 oz black olives, 2 sweet peppers, 2 large tomatoes, 1 cucumber, and 1 cup crumbled feta in a dressing of 6 tbsp olive oil, 1 tsp dried oregano, and a dash of pepper. Share half with a friend worthy of it!

### Afternoon Snack

Sweet-Baked Banana
TL;DR Toss two ripe, sliced bananas in 4 tsp honey and ¾ tsp cinnamon. Bake on a lined baking sheet at 350F for 10-15 minutes. Split half with a friend worthy of it!

### Dinner

Spanish Seafood Fried Rice

TL;DR Fry ¼ cup minced onion, ¼ cup diced sweet pepper, and 1 clove minced garlic in ½ tbsp olive oil over medium heat until tender. Add 1 cup instant brown rice, 2/3 cup vegetable broth, ¼ tsp thyme, a dash of saffron, and a dash of pepper. Once boiling, cover until vegetable broth evaporates. Add 8 oz shrimp, ½ cup peas, and arrange 8 oz mussels in a layer over top. Steam until mussels open. Remove from heat and let stand until vegetable broth is soaked up. Eat ½ today and save the rest for Saturday's dinner.

**Nutrient Breakdown**

Calories – 1301
Fat in grams – 46
Carbs in grams – 153
Fiber in grams – 25
Protein in grams – 54

# Friday

## Breakfast

Half of the Good Morning Couscous from Wednesday's breakfast.

## Mid-morning Snack

½ cup plain low-fat Greek yoghurt topped with ½ cup raspberries and 1 tsp honey.

## Lunch

Last remaining portion of Greek-Style Couscous from Tuesday's lunch.

## Afternoon Snack

Baguette topped with Feta Cheese and Olives Marinade leftover from Wednesday's mid-morning snack.

## Dinner

Reheat the remaining portion of Wednesday's Vegetarian Pasta Bolognese.

## Nutrient Breakdown

Calories – 1757
Fat in grams – 90
Carbs in grams – 220
Fiber in grams – 31
Protein in grams – 83

# Saturday

## Breakfast

Spanish Omelet
TL;DR Whisk together 4 eggs, ¼ cup low-fat milk, ½ diced tomato, 1 tbsp chopped chives, and a dash of pepper. Cook over medium heat and slowly crumble in 1 oz goat cheese. Place in an oven preheated to 375F for 9 minutes. Split in half and share with a friend.

## Mid-morning Snack

Ten almonds and ten grapes (frozen grapes are awesome).

## Lunch

Pulse ½ cup low-fat Greek yoghurt, ½ cup strawberries, ¼ cup low-fat milk, 1 tsp honey, and a dash of cinnamon in a blender to create a smoothie.

## Afternoon Snack

Sliced red sweet pepper with ¼ cup Spicy Red Pepper Spread to Dip.

## Dinner

Reheat Spanish Seafood Fried Rice from Thursday's dinner.

## Nutrient Breakdown

Calories – 1037
Fat in grams – 44
Carbs in grams – 99
Fiber in grams – 13
Protein in grams – 41

# Chapter 7 – Adjusting the Meal Plan

I would like to mention that if you're making adjustments to suit your nutrition needs, not every single adjustment listed needs to be used. For example, if you needed to add a couple hundred more calories but followed through with all my suggestions for adding calories, you will most likely end up way over your calorie count. Instead, pick and choose 1-3 of the ones which sound the most appetizing. And don't forget, a glass of wine at dinner is encouraged! Here's to eating great food, optimizing your health, and embracing the Mediterranean way of life!

## Sunday

### For less calories

Eliminate maple syrup from Fluffy Mediterranean Pancakes. Have less Spicy Red Pepper Dip at your mid-morning snack. Eliminate shrimp from Seafood Pasta. Eliminate or have fewer walnuts at mid-afternoon snack. Eliminate olive oil from Italian Potato Salad and make the sauce by boiling it instead of frying it.

### For more calories

Make the yoghurt and milk from the Fluffy Mediterranean Pancakes 2%. Add whole-wheat toast to your mid-morning snack. Add more olive oil and/or shrimp to the Seafood Pasta. Have 10 walnuts instead of 5 at your afternoon snack. Add mayonnaise or more olive oil to Italian Potato Salad. Have a dessert after dinner (there are plenty great options in the 50 Scrumptious Recipes chapter).

### Still hungry?

Use more strawberries on your Fluffy Mediterranean Pancakes at breakfast. Eat a full cucumber at your mid-morning snack. Make a simple salad with your Seafood Pasta at lunch. Have some veggies or an extra orange at your afternoon snack. Use more cherry tomatoes in your Italian Potato Salad at dinner. Have some fruit for dessert after dinner.

## Monday

### For less calories

Use just a half-avocado or ¾ oz feta cheese with Green Eggs and Toast. Alternatively, you could also replace the egg with cucumber slices. Eliminate chicken or use less feta cheese in the Greek-Style Couscous. Have less or eliminate almonds from your afternoon snack. Use less or eliminate mozzarella and parmesan from the Cheesy Eggplant Sandwich.

### For more calories

Mash 1 tbsp olive oil into avocado for Green Eggs and Toast. Wrap each date in 2 slices prosciutto. Add more chicken or ½ cup grated mozzarella cheese to the Greek-Style Couscous. Add 3-4 olives to your afternoon snack. Double the cheese and/or spread 1 full tsp olive oil over bread for Cheesy Eggplant Sandwich. Have a dessert after dinner (there are plenty great options in the 50 Scrumptious Recipes chapter)

### Still hungry?

Put some tomato slices on your Green Eggs and Toast at breakfast. Have some veggies with your mid-morning snack. Add a diced cucumber to your Greek-Style Couscous at lunch. Add some veggies to your afternoon snack. Have a full cup of spinach with your Cheesy Eggplant Sandwich at dinner. Have some fruit for dessert after dinner.

## Tuesday

### For less calories

Eliminate maple syrup from Fluffy Mediterranean Pancakes. Have fewer or eliminate walnuts from your mid-morning snack. Eliminate shrimp from Seafood Pasta. Have less Spicy Red Pepper Dip at your afternoon snack. Eliminate olive oil from Italian Potato Salad and make the sauce by boiling it instead of frying it.

For more calories

Make the yoghurt and milk from the Fluffy Mediterranean Pancakes 2%. Add 5 more walnuts or 3-4 olives to your mid-morning snack. Add more olive oil and/or shrimp to the Seafood Pasta. Add whole-wheat toast to your afternoon snack. Add mayonnaise or more olive oil to Italian Potato Salad. Have a dessert after dinner (there are plenty great options in the 50 Scrumptious Recipes chapter)

Still hungry?

Use more strawberries on your Fluffy Mediterranean Pancakes at breakfast. Have another orange and/or some veggies with your mid-morning snack. Make a simple salad with your Seafood Pasta at lunch. Add a sliced carrot or some fruit to your afternoon snack. Use more cherry tomatoes in your Italian Potato Salad at dinner. Have some fruit for dessert after dinner.

## Wednesday

For less calories

Make the milk in your Good Morning Couscous low-fat milk and/or eliminate 1 tsp brown sugar topping. Use ¼ cup low-fat feta and/or 1 ½ tbsp olive oil in the Feta Cheese and Olives Marinade at your mid-morning snack. Eliminate chicken or use less feta cheese in the Greek-Style Couscous. Eliminate honey from your afternoon snack. Eliminate 5 oz beans from the Vegetarian Pasta Bolognese at dinner.

For more calories

Add 1 ½ tsp cinnamon to your Good Morning Couscous. Use full-fat feta and/or 1 tbsp olive oil in the Feta Cheese and Olive Marinade at your mid-morning snack. Add more chicken or ½ cup grated mozzarella cheese to the Greek-Style Couscous. Use full-fat Greek yoghurt for your afternoon snack. Add 1 tbsp olive oil to the Vegetarian Pasta Bolognese sauce. Have a dessert after dinner (there are plenty great options in the 50 Scrumptious Recipes chapter).

Still hungry?

Use more currants in your Good Morning Couscous. Have some veggies along with the Feta Cheese and Olive Marinade at your mid-morning snack. Add a diced cucumber to your Greek-Style Couscous at lunch. Use a full cup of blackberries on the yoghurt at your afternoon snack. Use more veggies in your Vegetarian Pasta Bolognese at dinner. Have some fruit for dessert after dinner.

**Thursday**

For less calories

Use only 1 tbsp granola in your Fruity Yoghurt Parfait. Have less Spicy Red Pepper Dip at your mid-morning snack. Use only ½ cup feta cheese and/or 3 tbsp olive oil in your Classic Greek Salad at lunch. Use only 3 tsp honey at your afternoon snack. Use less shrimp or mussels in the Spanish Seafood Fried Rice at dinner.

For more calories

Use full-fat yoghurt and/or more granola in your Fruity Yoghurt Parfait at breakfast. Add whole-wheat toast to your mid-morning snack. Use more olive oil and/or feta cheese in your Classic Greek Salad at lunch. Use 1 ½ cups instant brown rice in the Spanish Seafood Fried Rice at dinner. Have a dessert after dinner (there are plenty great options in the 50 Scrumptious Recipes chapter).

Still hungry?

Use more raspberries in your Fruity Yoghurt Parfait at breakfast. Have more carrots with your mid-morning snack or add some fruit. Use more tomatoes, sweet peppers, and/or cucumbers in your Classic Greek Salad at lunch. Have one more banana with your afternoon snack. Add more sweet pepper to your Spanish Seafood Fried Rice at dinner or serve a salad on the side. Have some fruit for dessert after dinner.

**Friday**

For less calories

Make the milk in your Good Morning Couscous low-fat milk and/or eliminate 1 tsp brown sugar topping. Eliminate honey from your mid-morning snack. Eliminate chicken or use less feta cheese in the Greek-Style Couscous. Use ¼ cup low-fat feta and/or 1 ½ tbsp olive oil in the Feta Cheese and Olives Marinade at your afternoon snack. Eliminate 5 oz beans from the Vegetarian Pasta Bolognese at dinner.

For more calories

Add 1 ½ tsp cinnamon to your Good Morning Couscous. Use 2% yoghurt at your mid-morning snack. Add more chicken or ½ cup grated mozzarella cheese to the Greek-Style Couscous. Use full-fat feta and/or 1 tbsp olive oil in the Feta Cheese and Olive Marinade at your afternoon snack. Add 1 tbsp olive oil to the Vegetarian Pasta Bolognese sauce. Have a dessert after dinner (there are plenty great options in the 50 Scrumptious Recipes chapter).

Still hungry?

Use more currants in your Good Morning Couscous. Use a full cup of raspberries in your Greek yoghurt at mid-morning snack. Add a diced cucumber to your Greek-Style Couscous at lunch. Have some veggies along with the Feta Cheese and Olive Marinade at your afternoon snack. Use more veggies in your Vegetarian Pasta Bolognese at dinner. Have some fruit for dessert after dinner.

## Saturday

### For less calories

Use ½ oz goat cheese in your morning Spanish Omelet. Eat less or eliminate almonds from your mid-morning snack. Eliminate honey from your smoothie at lunch. Have less Spicy Red Pepper Dip at your afternoon snack. Use less shrimp or mussels in the Spanish Seafood Fried Rice at dinner.

### For more calories

Use 2% milk in your morning Spanish Omelet. Add 3-4 olives to your mid-morning snack. Use 2% yoghurt and milk in your smoothie at lunch. Add whole-wheat toast to your afternoon snack. Use 1 ½ cups instant brown rice in the Spanish Seafood Fried Rice at dinner. Have a dessert after dinner (there are plenty great options in the 50 Scrumptious Recipes chapter).

### Still hungry?

Use a full tomato in your Spanish Omelet at breakfast and serve with a side of fruit. Add more grapes or some veggies to your mid-morning snack. Use a full cup of strawberries in your smoothie at lunch. Slice a cucumber to have along with the sweet pepper during your afternoon snack. Add more sweet pepper to your Spanish Seafood Fried Rice at dinner or serve a salad on the side. Have some fruit for dessert after dinner.

# Chapter 8 – Mediterranean Myths

As with any diet, the myths that are associated with it can lead to frustration, confusion, and failure. To ensure you don't run into these issues, I thought I'd dedicate a chapter to clearing up the muddy waters of the Mediterranean diet. These myths are the worst offenders, and I'm here to ensure you won't fall victim to their ways.

You can eat any and all food as long as it's Mediterranean – The Mediterranean diet is based on foods which are so nutrient rich that they can actually make you overweight if eaten in excess. For example, you can't expect to have a box of pasta doused in olive oil followed by a bottle of wine every night and lose weight. Unfortunately, this is a common misconception on the Mediterranean diet. No more than four tablespoons of olive oil or one glass of wine per day is recommended. At that point, it's just no longer a diet. Weight loss surgeon, Dr. Joseph J Colella, suggests that to be successful while on the Mediterranean diet one must strategically portion richer foods while indulging most in fresh foods such as fruits and vegetables. Moderation is the key to success on the Mediterranean diet.

Calorie counting is a waste of time – This point sort of goes along with the last in the way that if followed incorrectly, one can become massively obese while on the Mediterranean diet. Along with portion control, calorie counting is another important factor to success with the Mediterranean diet. It is especially important if your main reason for going on the Mediterranean diet is to lose weight. At the end of the day, the calories you ate versus the calories you worked off will determine your weight loss results. If you missed it, be sure to check out how to determine your daily calorie count in the What You'll Be Eating chapter.

Mediterranean food is cheap – If in the past, you purchased food for the sole reason that it was cheap, you will notice that your wallet will be considerably lighter when you switch to the

Mediterranean diet. This is arguably the worst side effect of the diet, but one which can't be avoided. Cost of food which is fresh and wholesome versus food which is processed and packaged is vastly different. For this reason, it's important that you take into account beforehand that your grocery budget will need to expand. You can easily keep your funds strong by making room in other ways, however. For example, since the Mediterranean diet strongly discourages smoking and heavy drinking, this money could instead go towards buying more wholesome, healthy foods.

It's just a diet - Many people who go on the Mediterranean diet believe that they will only need to change their eating habit. This is far from true, however, as the Mediterranean diet requires that you change many other aspects along with food. It's difficult to achieve most positive results on the diet if you don't fit in some moderate exercise as well. Sharing food with others and in a dining-room setting helps as well – it encourages healthy relationships, helps with portion control, and prevents mindless eating. These things may be considered just as good for your health as what you put in your mouth. To achieve all benefits from the Mediterranean diet, one has to think of it in a most universal way.

Wine is all you need – Water is the favored drink on the Mediterranean diet as it is calorie free and helps to flush our body of poisonous toxins. In fact, our body is comprised 60% of water, so it's especially important we drink enough of it to maintain a healthy body composition. Without drinking an adequate amount of water, we will become dehydrated, feel sluggish, and be unable to carry through with the most basic everyday tasks. The one thing that health professionals all over the world insist upon is that we stay hydrated – especially while starting a new diet or making a drastic lifestyle change. In general, the Mediterranean diet suggests that we drink at least 6 glasses of water per day. It is important to keep in mind, however, that each of our lifestyles and bodies are a little different, meaning that some of us will require more water than others.

Wine, wine, and more wine! –Many people assume that if one glass of wine is considered healthy, then the whole bottle must turn you into Superman! While this may be true mentally (although I do not encourage you to test that theory out!), it is certainly not true physically. Only moderate amounts of wine will produce unique benefits for your heart, while too much wine will only do considerable damage. As a rule of thumb, you should consume no more than one glass of wine per day if you're a woman and two glasses of wine per day if you're a man.

Dried fruit is just as good as fresh – Most dried fruit found in any supermarket around the world contains a scary amount of sulfites. Figures are not well defined as actual analyses are hard to come by, but it is estimated that the amount of sulfites in most dried fruit is at or above the specified limit for most adults (0.70 mg/Kg per kilogram of body weight). Dried apricots, peaches, and pears that were chemically analyzed showed to have an average sulfite level of 2885 mg/kg. To serve as comparison, the average hot dog showed to have just 8 mg.

Fruit juice counts as a serving of fruit – Most fruit juice you buy in the supermarket today does a lot more bad than good. While it is true that fruit juices contain very healthy vitamins and antioxidants, they just don't have enough to make up for the amount of sugar found in the drinks. In fact, most fruit juice has just as much or more sugar than your average can of coke. This means that even if you're drinking a juice labeled as "100% pure" or "not from concentrate", it doesn't mean it's particularly healthy. Let's take the standard process for making fruit juice into consideration, shall we? After the juice has been squeezed from the fruit, it is then put into a massive oxygen-depleted holding tank and stored for up until a year before it's even considered for packaging. Needless to say, the juice loses a lot of its flavor over this time, so the manufacturers compensate by adding "flavor packs" (basically lots of chemicals and sugar). In the end, the product that you end up drinking is really just fruit-flavored-sugar-water. Some of the worst offenders for this practice are Minute Maid, Ocean Spray, Santa Cruz Organic, Naked Juice, Simply Orange, Del Monte, V8, and Bolthouse Farms. There are, however, a few fruit juice brands that can be trusted. Some healthy brands include Natalie's Orchid Island Juice, Mott's Natural, Old Orchard Organics, Simply Grapefruit, Whole Foods 365, Tropicana Pure Valencia, Martinelli's Gold Medal, Pom, and RW Knudsen.

Salt your foods for flavor – Avoid salt at all costs and use herbs instead! One food ingredient which many end up eating far too much of is salt. It is especially important that you watch your sodium intake if you're trying to recover from high blood pressure. The Center for Disease Control and Prevention has stated that 77% of the sodium we consume comes from either processed foods or restaurant foods. This means that while on the Mediterranean diet, hidden sodium sources to watch out for will be breads, cold cuts, pizza, poultry, soups, sandwiches, cheese, pasta dishes, meat dishes, and various snacks. Some of these foods are obviously unavoidable as they are staples in the Mediterranean diet, but researchers believe the high sodium count is balanced out with adequate amounts of fruits, vegetables, and olive oil. That's why it's so important to keep an eye on how much you consume of these foods high in sodium – eating too much means no amount of fruits, vegetables, or olive oil will be able to combat it. It is suggested that one can effectively keep an eye on their sodium intake by keeping their foods as fresh, organic, and wholesome as possible (or as least processed as possible). Food containing lots of sodium that cannot be avoided should be eaten in as much moderation as possible. For example, a serving of 3-4 olives instead of, say, 10, is sufficient.

The new age Mediterranean diet – The diet outlined in this book is not to be confused with the diet that those in the Mediterranean region are living off of in this decade. If we ate as the people in the Mediterranean region eat now, we wouldn't receive many positive results. The reason being is that since the Seven Countries Study was conducted, the diet of the Mediterranean has taken a turn for the worst. Many of the highly processed foods responsible for the obesity rates in America have now been adopted by most the rest of the world. Today, the Mediterranean diet consists mostly of red meat, cheese, sweets, and sugary drinks or in other words, all the foods responsible for making the Western world obese. In fact, a study conducted by the Organization for Economic Cooperation and Developments found that there is now a larger amount of obese children living in Greece and Italy than there is living in the United States. Needless to say, the Mediterranean diet should not mimic in the slightest what Mediterranean's eat in this day and age, but rather what they were eating a few decades ago. Given this dramatic shift in diet, there is no question why so much confusion now surrounds how one should eat on the Mediterranean diet. Thankfully, this guide provides accurate information on the Old-School Mediterranean diet – the one which will give you countless health benefits and make you feel better than you may have ever thought possible.

# Epilogue

I hope the first chapter offered some insight to our world's history, and especially that of the beautiful Mediterranean region, from customs to traditions to culture. I hope the tips, tricks, and myths break the diet down into something you can chew on, literally! Don't be afraid to refer back to them if you feel you're ever stuck. This book should serve as a one-stop-shop to all of your dieting questions, needs, and struggles. Also, I hope you already have the mental toughness it will take to fight everyone off of the delicious recipes I've included... I believe that may be the most challenging parts of your journey!

All jokes aside, I hope this book has shown you how simple it is to live a life of health, vitality, energy, and happiness far from anything you've ever experienced before. With so many diets failing people and so few success stories today, my heart can only hope that this book will finally provide you with some answers. Whether it's your weight that you struggle to keep under control or a chronic illness such as cardiovascular disease, diabetes, or high blood pressure I am sure the Mediterranean diet will offer some salvation. If you put the effort into changing your life to suit the ways of the Mediterranean now, I'm sure you will only thank yourself for the remainder. Regardless of what your goals are on this diet, whether it's to change your looks or your life, I send my motivation and congratulations. This book was the first step, and the first step often takes the most willpower and determination.

# MEDITERRANEAN DIET COOKBOOK

105 Easy, Irresistible and Healthy Recipes for Weight Loss and Improved Quality of Life

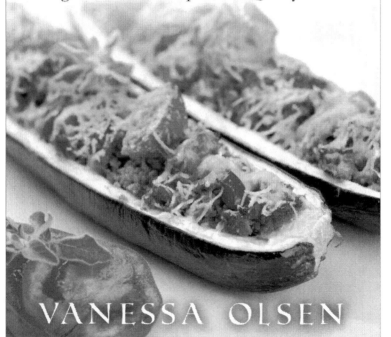

## VANESSA OLSEN

# Table of Contents

Introduction – More than a diet.

Chapter 1 – The History

Chapter 2 – Breakdown

Chapter 3 – Proven Benefits

Chapter 4 – Breakfast for Champions
- Crispy Breakfast Pitas
- On-the-Go Breakfast Wraps
- Veggie-licious Omelet
- Seaside Sunrise Sandwich
- Mediterranean Crockpot Breakfast
- Nutty for Greek Yoghurt
- Low-Cal Frittata
- Cinnamon Twisted Eggs
- Watermelon Salad
- Tomato and Olive Breakfast Pizza
- Honey Roasted Peaches
- Strawberry Crepes
- Couscous Oatmeal
- Walnut Strawberry Toast
- Peachy-Plum Parfait

Chapter 5 – 'Lax Lunches
- Greek-Style Egg Salad Sandwiches
- Vegetarian Grilled Cheese
- Zesty Orzo Salad
- Hearty Fish Casserole
- Cheesy Panini
- Creamy Chicken Enchiladas
- Cozy Kale Stew
- Gazpacho

- Feta Stuffed Quesadillas
- Collard Leaf Wraps
- Mediterranean Salad
- Mediterranean-Style Burger Patties
- Portside Tuna Salad
- Hummus Roll-Ups
- Simple Angel Hair Pasta

Chapter 6 – Dinner for Winners

- Baked Sweet Potatoes with Crunchy Chickpeas
- Oven Baked Cauliflower
- Zesty Lime Baked Chicken
- Savory Kale Spaghetti
- Shrimp on a Stick
- Tomato Layered Fish
- Tomato Eggplant Bake
- Tomato Patties
- Spicy Quinoa and Chickpea Salad
- Gluten-Free Zucchini Pizza
- Roasted Tomato Bowls
- Savory & Spicy Shrimp Spaghetti
- Tomato Basil Stuffed Peppers
- Veggie and Rice Casserole
- Onion Fried Eggs

Chapter 7 – Sides & Snacks

- Crispy Falafel
- Pita Crisps
- Zucchini Discs
- Spicy Potato Chunks
- Traditional Dolmades

Chapter 8 – Dips and Dollops

- Simple Tahini
- Mediterranean-Style Hummus
- Refreshing Tzatziki Sauce

- Traditional Mediterranean Aioli
- Lemon Caper Sauce
- Mediterranean-Style Salsa
- Dill Crazy Tartar Sauce
- Potato Skordalia
- Versatile Pesto
- Tapenade
- Spicy Cilantro Sauce
- Creamy Dill Sauce
- Greek Vinaigrette

Chapter 9 – Seaside Sippers

- Raspberry Fig Punch
- Citrus Sangria
- Raspberry Mojito with an Italian Twist
- Waterberry Sangria
- Lemonade Spritzer
- The Pink Lady
- Olive Devil
- Rose Petal Punch
- Mediterranean Adult Nestea
- Mediterranean Twisted Coffee

Chapter 10 – Delicious Desserts

- Walnut Crescent Cookies
- Traditional Ekmek Kataifi
- Flaky Coconut Pie
- Ricotta Cheese Fruit Bake
- Anginetti Lemon Cookies
- Toasted Almond Biscotti
- Greek Rice Pudding
- Doughnut Holes
- Sweet Ricotta-Filled Sandwiches
- Sesame Seed Crackers
- Avocado & Sweet Potato Cupcakes
- Spanish Fartons

- Classic Cannoli's
- Vasilopita Cake
- Honey Crisps

Epilogue

Bonus: FREE Paleo Diet Book

# Introduction – More than a diet.

In today's day and age, there is a lengthy list of diets which people can't adhere to for one main reason: it's just a diet! People will begin a diet with high hopes of improved health and better quality of life only to lose their way in a confusing set of guidelines and numbers. Sound familiar?

If it does, I'm *glad* a diet has failed you before. It only means you'll see the true worth of the Mediterranean diet – a diet which has little to do with number crunching and non-human eating strategies, but instead revolves around creating a life full of good food, healthy relationships, happiness, and longevity.

Indeed, the Mediterranean diet is about so much more than the kinds of foods you're eating. It comes as no surprise though, when we think about the lively, vibrant people who inhabit the Mediterranean region. Not only are their lives full, but they're healthy, too. And good health is one of the greatest blessings known to mankind.

And these people aren't healthy because they eat bird food day in and day out. These people are healthy because they've mastered the art of moderation. A little bit of this, a little bit of that, a little bit of love, and a little bit of fat. They create colorful, nutritious, and well balanced meals which contribute to their lives of ease and simplicity. It's all about focusing on getting the good stuff in us, and mixing it with little bits of indulgence. And that's exactly what this cookbook is about, too.

Upon flipping through the pages of this book you will encounter recipes of all types – some savory, some nutritious, yet all of them delicious. This cookbook focuses on creating a healthy lifestyle focused on spending time with loved ones and living every day to the fullest, just as the people of the Mediterranean region do best.

Not only are the recipes in this book absolutely delicious, but as the title reads, they will also result in some pretty amazing health benefits. I touch on those within the next couple of chapters, and if you can start to embrace the Mediterranean way of life, you can expect to reap those same benefits!

Welcome to the wonderful world of olive oil, feta cheese, seafood, and of course, wining and dining!

# Chapter 1 – The History

The Mediterranean diet came together as a result of sharing and exploring different cultures and traditions. This chapter goes over how all the bits of the Mediterranean diet came together. It's a story of life, love, and human connection.

The earliest form of the Mediterranean diet came about between 753BC and 476AD. It was the diet of the Ancient Romans and Egyptians. The people of these times, archaeologists conclude, had an impressively broad food palette. Not only that, but they treated food as a means of connecting people. Everything from gathering the food to making the food to eating the food was considered to be a social experience. Needless to say, their lives almost revolved around the topic of food entirely.

Evidence leftover in the form of tools and scribes tells us that the wealthy dined on a diet comprised mostly of breads, olive oil, and wines. Cheese and vegetables were also present, but not a priority since they were "...considered to be beneath the dignity of gods and heroes". Only trace amounts of meat were found in their diets, with chicken and seafood being about the only types of meat these people ever ate.

It was also between the years of 753BC and 476AD that the Arabian and Roman people began to delve into each other's cultures. The Arabians brought with them sugar, spice, rice, spinach, eggplant, pomegranate, rose water, almonds, and citrus fruit. The Romans were indeed very keen on this food, and because of this these foods are still widely used in the Mediterranean diet today.

After the clash of the Arabians and Romans, the Mediterranean diet slowed to a standstill. Nothing was changed or altered for many generations until 1492, when the brave Christopher Columbus set out to prove that the world was indeed not flat, but round. On his trip he discovered America, which again introduced new foods to the people of the Mediterranean. Now they were also dining on potatoes, beans, peppers, corn, cereals, chili, and tomatoes. The people of the Mediterranean were quite fond of these new additions, which is why they also have stuck around in the diet to date.

The Mediterranean ate and lived on in happy, normal fashion thinking nothing of their diet until the year of 1950, when people began to realize that there was something special about the foods they were eating. It was Ancel Keys, American Scientist, who first made the connection between food and our cardiovascular health. In order to prove his assumptions, he escaped to Italy to make a journal of the foods which these incredibly healthy people ate. He found that while the people of this region ate mostly pastas, veggies, and seafood, the people of the Western world were eating a diet rich in dairy. He concluded that this dairy-rich diet must have something to do with why there was such an epidemic for cardiovascular disease in America.

Keys then went on to expand his study into the "Seven Countries Study" which included the likes of Finland, Holland, Italy, the USA, Greece, Japan, and Yugoslavia. The results really changed the way our people look at food, and so much so the study sparked a sort of Mediterranean trend. Anyone who wanted to live a healthier life changed their diet to that of the Mediterranean and experienced some amazing results.

This Mediterranean trend still exists today (buying this book means even you're a part of it!) and for good reason. Eating traditional Mediterranean food has proved not only in the Seven Countries Study but in many more studies to provide some amazing health benefits. The next chapter will detail exactly how you can reap these benefits for yourself.

# Chapter 2 - Breakdown

So, what food does this flavorful diet come down to, you must be dying to know. Unfortunately, it's not about eating an endless amount of feta cheese and oil-soaked olives. Contrary to popular belief, it's not about eating copious amounts of pasta drizzled in a cream sauce either. But, it is about 3 main and absolutely delicious macronutrients:

*Carbs, fat, and protein.*

And yes, that list is in order from biggest to smallest.

To be exact, you will aim to consume 55-60% of your calories in the form of carbs, 25-30% of your calories in the form of fats, and 15-20% of your calories in the form of protein.

In our day and age, it seems that everyone fears carbs and fats. Maybe they're even the first things you look for when reading a nutrition label. If they are, it's time you stopped living like that, and started embracing them instead.

There's such thing as good carbs and bad carbs. There's also such thing as good fats and bad fats. While on the Mediterranean diet, you will be doing your best to consume (you guessed it...) the "good guys". For carbs, these are foods like vegetables, beans, oats, and grains. For fats, these are foods like avocados, cheese, dark chocolate, and whole eggs. I hope you're starting to see that the Mediterranean diet isn't so much a "diet" after all...

Apart from carbs, fats, and protein, the Mediterranean diet is mostly about keeping everything as well balanced and as nutritious as possible. Some foods in particular which are recommended include fruit, olive oil, and red wine. Hold up – what was that last part?!

Yes, as you may have already heard red wine is a big part of the Mediterranean way of life. It is obviously not recommended in excess though. For the ladies, 1 glass along with dinner is the recommendation, and for men, no more than 2.

While drinking wine is awesome, the best part about the Mediterranean diet is that *nothing* is off limits. The people of the Mediterranean region are very lively, genuine people. They're not about boycotting certain foods just to maintain a nice physique or even for the sake of health. Instead they're about eating all foods with emphasis on the good stuff and a strict moderation approach towards the bad stuff.

Along with the food component, however, also comes a complete lifestyle. Being on the Mediterranean diet is not just about what you're eating, but also how you're living. The people of the Mediterranean region recommend we cook and eat together, or in other words, turn food into a social experience. It's good for our mental health, which means it's good for our health overall.

Additionally, one long walk per day or a short workout at the gym a couple of times a week is also a part of the Mediterranean way of life. Some moderate exercise here and there is vital to keep everything running in tip-top shape, and this is exactly what the Mediterranean diet will do for you.

The next chapter goes over some health benefits you will experience while on the Mediterranean diet along with studies which prove they're legit. If you ever feel yourself slipping back into bad habits, give it a quick read. The thought of being in good health is quite arguably the best motivation known to mankind.

# Chapter 3 – Proven Benefits

The list of benefits that come with the Mediterranean diet could stretch on for miles, but for your benefit, I'll keep the list down to the main ones. In order to prove that the Mediterranean diet is a legit method to gain superior health, I've listed each benefit with a study which proves it to be true.

Prevention of Cardiovascular Disease – A study published by The New England Journal of Medicine had 7447 patients with high risk of developing cardiovascular disease prescribed to one of three diets: an olive oil-based Mediterranean diet, a mixed nut-based Mediterranean diet, and a control diet of reduced dietary fat. The trial continued for close to 5 years, leading researchers involved to conclude that a Mediterranean diet based on either olive oil or nuts had great effects on reducing the occurrence of major cardiovascular upset.

Weight Loss – Researchers at Mary Ann Liebert Inc. delved into the studies of the Mediterranean diet published by PubMed, Embase, and the Cochrane Central Register of Controlled Trials. To be exact, sixteen randomized controlled trials with over 5000 people involved were taken into account. The researchers concluded that most all participants on the Mediterranean diet had experienced significant weight loss, and especially when physical activity was involved or when the diet spanned longer than 6 months.

Prevention of Type 2 Diabetes – The American Diabetes Association published a study which had 418 non-diabetic subjects age 55-80 partake in the Mediterranean way of life. At the 4 year follow up, it appeared that those on the Mediterranean diet were a staggering 52% less likely to develop diabetes than those on the traditional American diet. The researchers concluded the diet by stating that the Mediterranean diet is in fact an effective method for the prevention of diabetes.

As you can see, we fitness gurus aren't just talking this diet up for the sake of it... Yet while these studies prove some truly amazing effects of the Mediterranean diet, these are only to name a few. The Mediterranean diet has also proven to be an effective method for prevention of stroke, high blood pressure, Alzheimer's, Parkinson's, and even cancer. That being said, this diet will not only change your life, but it may even *save* your life.

# Chapter 4 – Breakfast for Champions

## Crispy Breakfast Pitas (makes 2 servings)

Who would have ever thought that a pita would be a great way to start the day? These are as nutritious as they are delicious, with sautéed veggies and eggs to keep you up and running well into lunch time.

Ingredients:
2 tostadas
¼ cup red pepper, chopped
¼ cup hummus
¼ cup tomatoes, chopped
¼ cup cucumber, chopped
¼ cup green onions, minced
¼ cup milk
4 eggs
2 tablespoons feta cheese, crumbled
¼ teaspoon oregano
¼ teaspoon garlic powder

Directions:
1. Put a non-stick skillet with the red peppers over medium heat and stir occasionally for 2-3 minutes or until tender.
2. While the peppers cook, beat the eggs together until bubbly.
3. Once the peppers are tender, add the green onions, milk, eggs, oregano, and garlic powder to the skillet.
4. Stir the mixture constantly until eggs are fully cooked.
5. Once eggs are cooked and all ingredients are well combined, take the skillet off the heat and set aside.
6. Divide the hummus between the two tostadas and spread a nice, even layer on each.
7. Top each tostada with an even amount of the egg mixture, and garnish with the tomatoes and feta.
8. Plate and serve while warm!

Nutrient Breakdown (per one serving):
Calories – 328
Fat in grams – 18
Carbs in grams – 23
Fiber in grams – 4
Protein in grams – 20

## On-the-Go Breakfast Wraps (makes 8 wraps)

I call these "On-the-Go" because that's exactly the purpose they serve for me! I usually make them in large quantities and then freeze them for up to a month, grabbing one and simply giving it a 1-minute nuke on my busiest mornings. Not only do they save my life, but they're also incredibly delicious!

Ingredients:
8 whole wheat tortillas
2 cups spinach leaves, minced
½ cup canned tomatoes, drained and diced
½ cup feta cheese, crumbled
8 eggs
2 slices prosciutto, sliced thin
2 tablespoons milk
1 tablespoon olive oil
1 teaspoon garlic powder
Dash of pepper

Directions:
1. Whisk the eggs, milk, garlic powder, and pepper together in a medium-sized bowl until ingredients are well combined and mixture is bubbly.
2. Put a large skillet with the olive oil over medium heat.
3. Once oil is hot, add the egg mixture, stirring occasionally until eggs are cooked.
4. While the eggs cook, lay out the tortillas on a flat surface nearby.

5. Once the eggs are cooked, sprinkle them in a straight line over the tortillas. Make sure to divide this evenly as you go!
6. Divide the spinach, tomatoes, feta cheese, and prosciutto between the wraps, sprinkle them overtop the eggs.
7. Fold and roll! If you're not sure how, refer to this diagram.
8. Spray the skillet with cooking oil and press the wraps into them with a spatula. Keep them pressed until it seems that the tortillas have set and won't unwrap on you.
9. Eat one now and wrap the rest up for later! Roll them in some wax or parchment paper and stuff them into a large freezer bag.
10. Nuke as needed for the remainder of the month!

Nutrient Breakdown (per one wrap):
Calories – 238
Fat in grams – 11
Carbs in grams – 22
Fiber in grams – 3
Protein in grams – 15

# Veggie-licious Omelet (makes 2 servings)

This omelet is filled to the brim with delicious veggies that make the start of your day a healthy one. Add some crumbled feta cheese to make it a little more indulgent or serve with some whole wheat toast and fruit for a more balanced, filling meal.

Ingredients:
¼ cup + 2 tablespoons olive oil, divided
1 cup spinach, minced
½ cup onion, minced
½ cup bell pepper, chopped
¼ cup basil, minced
4 eggs

Directions:

1. Put a non-stick skillet with the 2 tablespoons olive oil over medium heat.
2. Once the oil is hot, add the spinach, onion, and bell pepper, stirring occasionally until veggies become tender.
3. Once the veggies are tender, transfer them to a bowl and set aside.
4. Crack the eggs into a bowl and whisk until bubbly.
5. Put the remaining olive oil in the skillet over medium-low heat and stir it around to give the skillet a good coating.
6. Pour in the eggs and let sit.
7. Once the bottom side of the eggs begins to set, sprinkle the veggies over one half of the omelet.
8. Carefully – *very* carefully – lift the edges of the omelet with a spatula. Then, dig the spatula in a little deeper on the veggie-free side and lift it up and over the side with the veggies.
9. Let the omelet cook for another 2 minutes before removing it from the pan.
10. Chop it in half, divide it between two plates, garnish with basil, and enjoy!

Nutrient Breakdown (per one serving):

Calories – 536
Fat in grams – 51
Carbs in grams – 7
Fiber in grams – 2
Protein in grams – 14

# Seaside Sunrise Sandwich (makes 2 sandwiches)

Say that title 10x fast! Not only is it a mouthful to say, but it's also a delicious mouthful to chew. All you salmon lovers out there – this one's for you!

Ingredients:
4 ounces smoked salmon, sliced
6 slices cucumber
2 whole wheat English muffins
2 slices red onion
2 tablespoons cream cheese
2 teaspoons capers, rinsed and drained

Directions:
1. Toast the English muffins to your preference
2. Spread the cream cheese on two halves of the English muffins.
3. Top the cream cheese with salmon, cucumber, red onion rings, and capers. Make sure to divide the ingredients evenly as you go!
4. Finish the sandwich by closing them up with their untouched halves.
5. Serve with some cherry tomatoes and lemon water and enjoy!

Nutrient Breakdown (per one sandwich):
Calories – 243
Fat in grams – 6
Carbs in grams – 25
Fiber in grams – 2
Protein in grams – 18

## Mediterranean Crockpot Breakfast (makes 3 servings)

Crockpots are awesome, but many overlook the fact that they're awesome for making breakfast, too! This recipe is perfect for lazy Sunday mornings and can easily feed a crowd if doubled.

Ingredients:
1 cup spinach, minced
½ cup feta cheese, crumbled
½ cup milk

½ cup Heart Healthy Bisquick
¼ cup sundried tomatoes, drained and diced
5 mini breakfast sausages, chopped
3 egg whites
1 egg
½ teaspoon garlic, minced
Dash of pepper
Dash of basil, minced

Directions:
1. Prep your crockpot by giving it a light coating of olive oil.
2. Whisk together the milk, Heart Healthy Bisquick, egg whites, and eggs in a medium-sized bowl until well combined.
3. Transfer mixture into slow cooker.
4. Sprinkle the spinach, feta, tomatoes, sausage, and garlic into the slow cooker. Stir this in with the egg mixture until well combined.
5. Cover your crockpot with its lid and let it do its thing on high heat for about two hours or until sides have browned slightly.
6. Spoon the finished quiche, dividing evenly, into 3 bowls.
7. Serve and enjoy!

Nutrient Breakdown (per one serving):
Calories – 263
Fat in grams – 16
Carbs in grams – 12
Fiber in grams – 3
Protein in grams – 50

## Nutty for Greek Yoghurt (makes 2 servings)

While there's not much to throwing this one together, it's packed with healthy fats, carbs, and proteins to keep you going on a busy day. Feel free to switch out the berries and nuts to whatever it is you have at home. There are so many creative possibilities!

Ingredients:
2 cups Greek yoghurt, low-fat
1 cup pecans, crushed
1 cup blackberries
2 tablespoons honey

Directions:
1.  Plop one cup of Greek yoghurt into two separate bowls.
2.  Mix ½ cup pecans and ½ cup blackberries into each.
3.  Top with the honey (divided evenly).
4.  Serve with your fanciest spoons and enjoy!

Nutrient Breakdown (per one serving):
Calories – 796
Fat in grams – 43
Carbs in grams – 66
Fiber in grams – 10
Protein in grams – 15

## Low-Cal Frittata (makes 3 servings)

This one is so filling, it's kind of hard to believe that it's really as low-cal as it is. Whenever I've got a night of wining and dining ahead of me, this recipe is my go-to to compensate for those calories. Not to mention, it's quite the savory dish.

Ingredients:
8 egg whites
2 cups spinach
½ cup feta cheese, crumbled
2 tablespoons olive oil
1 green pepper, seeds removed and chopped
1 red pepper, seeds removed and chopped
¼ medium onion, minced
1 teaspoon pepper

Directions:
1. Preheat oven to 375 degrees Fahrenheit.
2. Put a heavy skillet with the olive oil over medium-low heat.
3. Once the oil is hot, add in the green pepper, red pepper and onion, stirring occasionally until soft.
4. Sprinkle the pepper overtop somewhere in between the softening process.
5. Once the veggies have softened, add the egg whites and let sit for about 3 minutes or until cooked.
6. Sprinkle the feta cheese and spinach leaves overtop.
7. Transfer the skillet to the oven and let bake for 8-10 minutes or until spinach has wilted.
8. Remove skillet from the oven (be sure to wear an oven mitt!).
9. Loosen the edges of the frittata with a spatula before slicing it into 3 pieces.
10. Divide the pieces amongst 3 plates, serve, and enjoy!

Nutrient Breakdown (per serving):
Calories – 200
Fat in grams – 14
Carbs in grams – 8
Fiber in grams – 3
Protein in grams – 14

# Cinnamon Twisted Eggs (makes 2 servings)

Sweet, creamy, and savory... this unexpected combo sure makes for a mouth-watering meal. It's as easy as chopping everything up and throwing it in the oven to do its thing. Needless to say, I often put it together on those care-free Saturday mornings.

Ingredients:
4 eggs
6 slices Romano cheese
½ can (or 14 ounces) whole tomatoes, drained and chopped
1 small onion, minced

1 garlic clove, minced
1 tablespoon olive oil
¼ teaspoon sugar
¼ teaspoon cinnamon
¼ teaspoon red pepper flakes
1/8 teaspoon allspice
1/8 teaspoon cloves
Dash of pepper

Directions:
1. Preheat oven to 400 degrees Fahrenheit.
2. Put a medium-sized pot with the olive oil over medium heat.
3. Once the oil is hot, add the onions and let cook until tender.
4. Add in the garlic and let cook until fragrant.
5. Add in the tomatoes, sugar, cinnamon, red pepper flakes, allspice, and pepper, stirring until all ingredients are well combined.
6. Turn the heat down to low and let the mixture simmer for about 10 minutes, or until tomatoes break down.
7. Divide the mixture between 2 heat-proof bowls and crack the 2 eggs over top of each.
8. Place the bowls in the oven and let bake for 15 minutes or until the whites set. Turn the dishes halfway through.
9. Top each dish with 3 slices of Romano cheese, let that melt in, and enjoy!

Nutrient Breakdown (per one serving):
Calories – 592
Fat in grams – 40
Carbs in grams – 16
Fiber in grams – 3
Protein in grams – 42

# Watermelon Salad (makes 2 servings)

I *love* starting my mornings off with some fresh fruit, and this recipe gives me perfect opportunity to do so! This is definitely a favorite in my household, and especially in the summer as this is when the local watermelon is in its prime!

Ingredients:
40 cherry tomatoes, halved
4 slices watermelon, diced with rinds removed
1 cup feta cheese, crumbled
½ medium cucumber, diced
1 tablespoon olive oil
½ tablespoon balsamic vinegar
½ tablespoon mint, minced
Dash of pepper

Directions:
1. Put the olive oil, balsamic vinegar, mint, and pepper in a small jar and shake until well combined.
2. Put the cherry tomatoes, watermelon, feta cheese, and cucumber in a medium-sized bowl. Gently toss until all ingredients are well distributed.
3. Pour the dressing over top the salad and give it another gentle toss until the entire salad has an even coating.
4. Divide the salad between two bowls, serve, and enjoy!

Nutrient Breakdown (per one serving):
Calories – 427
Fat in grams – 20
Carb in grams – 60
Fiber in grams – 10
Protein in grams – 56

## Tomato and Olive Breakfast Pizza (makes 5 servings)

If anyone has ever told you that you shouldn't have pizza for breakfast, you should stop talking to them. No one needs that kind of negativity in their life! Here's a recipe which makes pizza for breakfast something both nutritious and delicious. Feeding a crowd has never been so easy!

Ingredients:
1 readymade whole-wheat pizza dough
¾ cup feta cheese, crumbled
¼ cup milk
¼ cup whole-wheat flour
1 medium tomato, diced
½ bell pepper, chopped
4 eggs
6 black olives, chopped
2 green onions, minced
2 tablespoons ranch dressing, reduced-fat
1 tablespoon olive oil
Dash of pepper

Directions:
1. Preheat oven to 475 degrees Fahrenheit.
2. In a medium-sized bowl, whisk together the eggs, milk, and pepper until well combined and bubbly. Set aside.
3. Put a non-stick pan with the olive oil over medium heat.
4. Once the oil is hot, add the bell pepper and let cook until tender.
5. Once the bell pepper is soft, pour in the egg mixture and stir until eggs are cooked through. Set aside.
6. Dust the flour over a pizza stone and stretch your pizza dough out over it.
7. Using your fingers, pinch together 1 inch of the parameter to create your pizza's crust.
8. Spoon and spread the ranch dressing over the pizza dough, avoiding the crust, of course.
9. Sprinkle the egg mixture evenly over the pizza dough. Finish off with the crumbled feta cheese, tomatoes, black olives, and green onions. Make a pretty picture, distribute it randomly – it's up to you!
10. Place the pizza in the oven and let it bake for 15 minutes or until the dough has risen and the crust is a light-brown color.
11. Remove pizza from the oven and let it cool for a couple minutes.
12. Divide it into 10 slices, place 2 on each plate, and enjoy!

Nutrient Breakdown (per one serving):
Calories – 419
Fat in grams – 16
Carbs in grams – 60
Fiber in grams – 5
Protein in grams – 18

## Honey Roasted Peaches (makes 2 servings)

This recipe is a sweet start to the day – that's for sure! The honey works its way into the peaches, sweetening them beyond compare while the pistachios add an unexpected dimension. It's sure to be a hit amongst adults and kids alike.

Ingredients:
2 large peaches, diced
¼ cup honey
¼ cup pistachios, chopped
Dash of caster sugar

Directions:
1. Put a non-stick pan with the peaches, honey, pistachios, and caster sugar over medium heat.
2. Let cook, stirring occasionally, for about 10-minutes so that the flavors can pull through the peaches.
3. Remove from heat and divide the mixture between 2 bowls.
4. Serve on top or with a side of Greek yoghurt and enjoy!

Nutrient Breakdown (per one serving):
Calories – 280
Fat in grams – 8
Carbs in grams – 54
Fiber in grams – 4
Protein in grams – 5

## Strawberry Crepes (makes 2 crepes)

I can remember my mother cooking crepes since I was young enough to roll them up myself! We used to have them for breakfast, lunch, and dinner, experimenting with different nutritious fillings and flavors. This strawberry recipe is one I hold close to my heart... mostly because it's just *so* sweet and savory.

Ingredients:
20 strawberries, diced
2 ounces cream cheese
1/3 cup whole wheat flour
1/3 cup milk
1 egg
1 tablespoon olive oil
1 teaspoon Stevia

Directions:
1. In a medium-sized bowl, stir together the strawberries and ½ teaspoon of Stevia until well combined. Set aside.
2. In another medium-sized bowl, whisk together the flour, milk, egg, and olive oil until bubbly. Set aside.
3. Take 1/3 of the strawberries and drop them in a blender with the cream cheese. Pulse until smooth. This will be your strawberry sauce. Set it aside for later.
4. Spray a pan with cooking spray and set it over medium-high heat.
5. Once the pan is hot, pour in ½ of the crepe batter.
6. Immediately begin tilting the pan so that the crepe covers the entire surface of it. *Tip: You have to move quickly otherwise your crepes will come out far too thick!*
7. Let the crepe cook for 45 seconds to 1 minute on the first side, then flip it and allow it to cook for another 20 seconds on the other side.
8. Once the crepe has pretty light brown dots and patterns on both sides, you'll know it's done. Set it aside and repeat steps 5-7 with the remaining batter.

9. Divide the strawberry sauce from before between the two crepes, spreading it in a nice even layer over both.
10. Divide the strawberries between the two crepes, assembling them in a straight line down the middle. Tip: You may want to leave some strawberries to garnish.
11. Pierce a fork parallel to the line of strawberries and roll the crepe up gently.
12. Top the crepes with the remaining strawberries, serve, and enjoy!

Nutrient Breakdown (per one crepe):
Calories – 321
Fat in grams – 19
Carbs in grams – 27
Fiber in grams – 4
Protein in grams – 10

# Couscous Oatmeal (makes 2 servings)

This Mediterranean alternative to oatmeal is unbelievably sweet and creamy yet still has all the vitamins and minerals you look for in a well-balanced meal. Usually I'll put this in a thermos and take it to work with me, but only on the days I feel like batting my co-workers away from it!

Ingredients:
1 cup water
½ cup milk
½ cup couscous
¼ cup dates, chopped
2 tablespoons honey
¼ teaspoon cinnamon

Directions:
1. Put the water and milk in a pot over high heat and bring to a boil.

2. Once the pot is boiling, add in the couscous, dates, and cinnamon. Cover and let cook for 5 minutes or until couscous in cooked through.
3. Divide between two bowls and drizzle 1 tablespoon honey over each.
4. Serve with a side of fresh fruit and enjoy!

Nutrient Breakdown (per serving):
Calories – 260
Fat in grams – 2
Carbs in grams – 53
Fiber in grams – 4
Protein in grams – 8

# Walnut Strawberry Toast (makes 2 servings)

If you already have the walnut butter on hand this one is an absolute breeze to put together. Feel free to switch out the bread for whole wheat and change the berries to whatever you have on hand. I've tried a couple variations and they're all equally delicious!

Ingredients:
4 pieces sourdough bread
¼ cup walnut butter
10 strawberries, sliced
6 thyme leaves
2 tablespoons honey

Directions:
1. Toast sourdough bread to your preference.
2. Divide and spread walnut butter over bread.
3. Top with strawberries and thyme leaves.
4. Drizzle with honey.
5. Plate and serve with some lemon water!

Nutrient Breakdown (per one serving):
Calories – 425
Fat in grams – 21

Carbs in grams – 52
Fiber in grams – 5
Protein in grams – 10

## Peachy-Plum Parfait (makes 2 servings)

Colossal layers of fruit, yoghurt, and walnuts explode over your taste buds as you devour this simple breakfast. I often prepare this one the night before an early, hectic morning by layering all the ingredients the night before and then adding the puffed cereal on the day of.

Ingredients:
2 cups plums, peaches, and nectarines, sliced
¾ cup puffed rice cereal
¾ cup plain Greek yoghurt, fat-free
2 tablespoons walnuts and almonds, toasted and halved
1 tablespoon honey
1 tablespoon flaxseed, ground

Directions:
1. Assemble two of your prettiest tall glasses.
2. Make alternate layers of fruit, cereal, yoghurt, nuts, flaxseed, and honey in each glass, dividing ingredients evenly as you go. You can be as creative and wild as you wish!
3. Eat with your fanciest long spoons and enjoy!

Nutrient Breakdown (per serving):
Calories – 225
Fat in grams – 6
Carbs in grams – 34
Fiber in grams – 5
Protein in grams – 11

# Chapter 5 – 'Lax Lunches

## Greek-Style Egg Salad Sandwiches (makes 2 sandwiches)

Here's a real classic with a refreshing Mediterranean twist. Greek yoghurt replaces the mayo in this recipe to create something a little more nutritious, while the diced cucumbers and sundried tomatoes maintain that delicious crunch and flavor.

Ingredients:
4 slices whole wheat bread
4 eggs, hardboiled
¼ cup red onion, minced
¼ cup sundried tomatoes, dried and chopped
¼ cup plain Greek yoghurt
2 tablespoons black olives, sliced
¼ cucumber, diced
1 teaspoon oregano
1/8 teaspoon cumin
Dash of pepper
Dash of lemon juice

Directions:
1. De-shell and dice up your hardboiled eggs, placing the bits in a bowl.
2. Ad in the red onion, sundried tomatoes, olives, and cucumber, gently tossing until ingredients are well combined.
3. Stir in the Greek yoghurt, oregano, cumin, pepper, and lemon juice until all ingredients are thoroughly incorporated.
4. Toast your bread to your preference.
5. Spread half the egg salad over one slice of toast, and the other half over another slice. Tip: Drizzle olive oil over

the toast before spreading on the egg salad if you want to create a richer flavor experience.
6. Close your sandwiches with the other slice of toast.
7. Plate and enjoy!

Nutrient Breakdown (per one sandwich):
Calories – 420
Fat in grams – 16
Carbs in grams – 47
Fiber in grams – 7
Protein in grams – 22

# Vegetarian Grilled Cheese (makes 2 sandwiches)

Grilled cheese has been one of my favorite dishes since I was a little girl. That being said, there's no way I could've given it up just because I went Mediterranean! When I first created this recipe I was pleasantly surprised as it tasted 10x better the tradition grilled cheese. I guess you'll just have to see for yourself though...

Ingredients:
4 ounces mozzarella cheese, sliced
2 ounces feta cheese, crumbled
4 cups spinach
¼ cup black olives, pitted and sliced
8 tomato slices
4 slices whole wheat bread
1 clove garlic, minced
2 tablespoons red onion, minced
2 tablespoons olive oil
1 tablespoon basil, minced
Dash of pepper

Directions:
1. Put a non-stick skillet with 2 teaspoon olive oil over medium-high heat.

2. Once the oil is hot, add the spinach and garlic and cook until tender. Then, remove it from heat.
3. Stir the basil into the skillet and set aside for later.
4. Divide the mozzarella and feta cheese between two slices of bread and spread on in an even layer.
5. Layer 4 tomatoes over each slice of cheesed-up bread.
6. Divide the spinach mixture and spoon it over each slice of cheesed-up bread.
7. Divide the olives and red onions and sprinkle it over each slice of cheesed-up bread.
8. Finish by sprinkling a bit of pepper over each, and closing the sandwich up with the untouched slices of bread.
9. Drizzle 1 teaspoon olive oil into the skillet and add in one sandwich.
10. Fry the sandwich over medium heat, carefully rotating once the first side turns a golden-brown.
11. Once both sides are crispy golden-brown, repeat steps 9 and 10 with the remaining sandwich.
12. Plate and serve!

Nutrient Breakdown (per one sandwich):
Calories – 559
Fat in grams – 45
Carbs in grams – 35
Fiber in grams – 5
Protein in grams – 24

# Zesty Orzo Salad (makes 4 servings)

Pasta salads are a staple in the Mediterranean diet. This one in particular is both zesty and refreshing, containing enough veggies and carbs to keep you full and satisfied until dinner. Often times, I'll prepare this on a Sunday afternoon so I can bring it to work for lunch for the remainder of the week.

Ingredients:
8 ounces orzo pasta
½ cup spinach, chopped

¼ cup basil, minced
¼ cup black olives, sliced
¼ cup feta cheese, crumbled
¼ cup balsamic vinegar
¼ cup olive oil
½ bell pepper, de-seeded and diced
½ tomato, diced
Dash of pepper

Directions:
1. Cook orzo according to package directions.
2. Once orzo is cooked, drain and rinse it in cold water before transferring it to a bowl to chill in the fridge.
3. Once the pasta has chilled, toss it with the spinach, basil, black olives, feta cheese, bell pepper, and tomatoes until all ingredients are well combined.
4. In a jar, shake up the balsamic vinegar, olive oil, and pepper until thoroughly incorporated. Then, pour this over the pasta and toss until the entire salad has a nice coating.
5. Divide salad between 4 bowls, serve, and enjoy!

Nutrient Breakdown (per one serving):
Calories – 251
Fat in grams – 4
Carbs in grams – 47
Fiber in grams – 3
Protein in grams – 9

# Hearty Fish Casserole (makes 4 servings)

Casseroles are that one dish where no matter what kind of health kick I'm on, I have to find a way to make them work. They're real comfort food, this Mediterranean version encompassing all qualities of creamy, filling, and nutritious.

Ingredients:
20 ounces halibut fillets
1lb small white potatoes, quartered

¼ cup parsley, minced
¼ cup black olives, pitted and sliced
2 bell peppers, de-seeded and sliced
2 tomatoes, cut into wedges
3 garlic cloves, minced
2 tablespoons lemon juice
2 tablespoons olive oil
¼ teaspoon pepper

Directions:
1. Preheat oven to 400 degrees Fahrenheit.
2. Grease a casserole dish with 1 tablespoon olive oil.
3. Distribute the potatoes and bell pepper slices across the bottom of the dish.
4. Sprinkle the pepper over top.
5. Place dish in the oven and bake for 35 minutes or until potatoes are soft. Tip: It helps if you give this dish a good stir every 10 minutes.
6. While this is doing its thing, season the fish with pepper.
7. Remove casserole dish from the oven and evenly distribute the fish fillets, garlic, black olives, and tomatoes over top.
8. Squeeze the lemon juice and drizzle the remaining olive oil over top.
9. Garnish with the parsley and stick the casserole dish back in the oven, this time baking it for 25 minutes or until fish is cooked and flaky.
10. Remove casserole dish from the oven, divide it between 4 plates, serve, and enjoy!

Nutrient Breakdown (per serving):
Calories – 272
Fat in grams – 8
Carbs in grams – 26
Fiber in grams – 4
Protein in grams – 26

# Cheesy Panini (makes 2 Panini's)

Panini's seem to be gaining some massive attention in the past couple of years – and for good reason! They're versatile, nutritious, and delicious. It's like a whole new level of grilled cheese!

Ingredients:
4 slices whole grain bread
7 ounces roasted red peppers, sliced
¼ cup mayo
2 slices mozzarella cheese
½ zucchini, sliced thin
2 tablespoons olive oil
2 tablespoons basil leaves, minced
1 tablespoon black olives, pitted and chopped

Directions:
1. In a small bowl, mix together the mayo and basil leaves until well combined.
2. Spread this mayo-basil sauce over your whole wheat bread slices.
3. On two of the slices, layer the mozzarella cheese slices, zucchini, and roasted red peppers. Tip: Be sure to divide the ingredients evenly over the bread as you go.
4. Close the sandwiches by squishing the non-vegged slices over top, mayo side down.
5. Spread the olive oil over the outer sides of the sandwich bread.
6. Transfer your Panini's to a large non-stick pan and fry them over medium heat.
7. Once the sandwiches are a crispy, golden-brown on one side, flip them until crisp on the other side.
8. Plate, serve, and enjoy!

Nutrient Breakdown (per one Panini):
Calories – 489
Fat in grams – 33
Carbs in grams – 40
Fiber in grams – 7

Protein in grams – 10

# Creamy Chicken Enchiladas (makes 4 enchiladas)

If you're new to the world of enchiladas, all I have to say is that your world is about to be changed. Welcome to the world of ooey-gooey cheesy baked wraps, the kind that requires a fork and knife!

Ingredients:
4 whole wheat tortillas
1 ½ cups chicken, cooked and shredded
1 cup chicken broth
1 cup cheese of your choice, shredded
½ cup Greek yoghurt
½ bell pepper, de-seeded and chopped
1 tablespoon olive oil
1 ½ tablespoons whole wheat flour
1 ½ tablespoons butter
½ tablespoon parsley, minced
½ teaspoon Italian seasoning
Dash of pepper

Directions:
1. Preheat oven to 425 degrees Fahrenheit.
2. Spray your casserole dish down with some cooking spray.
3. Put a ½ tablespoon of olive oil in a pan over medium heat and add the shredded chicken. Let this cook until heated through.
4. Remove the pan from heat and add your shredded cheese. Stir this in until well incorporated.
5. Lay your tortillas out on a flat surface and divide the chicken-cheese mixture amongst them. You will create a straight line down the center of the tortillas.
6. Roll the tortillas up and place them seam-side-down in the casserole dish. Set aside for later.
7. Put the remaining olive oil in a pan over medium heat.

8. Once the oil is hot, add the peppers and cook, stirring occasionally for about 2 minutes or until soft.
9. Once the peppers are soft remove the pan from heat and set them aside.
10. Add in the butter and stir until melted in with the peppers.
11. Stir in the flour until well incorporated.
12. Add the chicken broth and whisk it in until the sauce thickens and is lump-free.
13. Stir in the Greek yoghurt and peppers until well combined.
14. Finish by seasoning with pepper, Italian seasoning, and half of the parsley. Mix these ingredients in until well combined.
15. Transfer this sauce to the casserole dish, pouring it over the tortillas.
16. Garnish with a little bit of extra shredded cheese... or a lot, depending on how cheeky you're feeling!
17. Place the casserole dish in the oven and let it bake for 20-25 minutes or until enchiladas are golden-brown and cheese is bubbly.
18. Remove casserole dish from the oven and let cool.
19. Garnish with the remaining parsley, serve, and enjoy!

Nutrient Breakdown (per one enchilada):
Calories – 338
Fat in grams – 18
Carbs in grams – 17
Fiber in grams – 4
Protein in grams – 28

# Cozy Kale Stew (makes 3 servings)

These are perfect on those cold, rainy days when you just want to curl up by the fire with a good book. Not to mention it's full of some awesome nutrition to keep your immunity up during the cold and flu season.

Ingredient:

16 ounces vegetable broth
7 ounces cannellini beans, drained and rinsed
2 cups kale, stems removed and chopped
½ cup farro
¼ cup parsley, stems intact
1 medium tomato, diced
1 medium carrot, diced
½ small onion, diced
1 stalk celery, chopped
2 garlic cloves, minced
1 bay leaf
1 tablespoon olive oil
½ tablespoon lemon juice
½ teaspoon oregano
Crumbled feta cheese, for garnish

Directions:
1. Put a pot with the oil over medium-high heat.
2. Once the oil is hot, add the carrots, onion, and celery and let cook for 3 minutes.
3. After 3 minutes, add the garlic and let cook until fragrant.
4. Once garlic is fragrant, pour in the vegetable broth, faro, tomatoes, bay leaf, and oregano, stirring until well combined.
5. Finally, dump in the parsley and leave it in a pile on top of the soup until it comes to a boil.
6. Once the soup is boiling, reduce the heat to medium-low and cover to cook for 10-15 minutes.
7. Spoon out as much parsley as you can and discard of it.
8. Out went the parsley, in goes the kale! Stir that stuff in real good and let cook for another 10 minutes.
9. At around the 8 minute mark, stir in the cannellini beans.
10. Once the kale and farro are tender, remove the bay leaf and divide the soup between 3 bowls.
11. Crumble some feta cheese on top and serve!

Nutrient Breakdown (per one serving):

Calories – 170
Fat in grams – 5
Carbs in grams – 28
Fiber in grams – 6
Protein in grams – 7

## Gazpacho (makes 2 servings)

This traditional tomato soup stands out for one reason – it's best served cold! If you're looking to add more protein, look no further than adding some shrimp. Crackers and cheese also make a great side with this one!

Ingredients:
2 cups tomatoes, diced
1/3 cup medium bell pepper, de-seeded and diced
¼ cup (+ extra for garnish) squishy whole wheat bread, torn and packed
¼ cup olive oil
1 small clove garlic, minced
½ tablespoon fresh cilantro, chopped
1 teaspoon sherry vinegar
Dash of cumin

Directions:
1. Put the tomatoes, bell peppers, torn bread, 3 tablespoons olive oil, garlic, sherry vinegar, and cumin in a blender and pulse until smooth. Tip: Be patient – this could take up to 5 minutes!
2. Put the mixture in the fridge and let it sit for one hour or until very cold.
3. While this mixture cools, put a skillet with the remaining olive oil over medium heat. Once the oil is hot, add a torn piece of bread. If it sizzles, add the rest of the pieces, too.
4. Stir the bread occasionally for about 1 minute or until golden brown.
5. Once the bread pieces are crispy and crouton-like, transfer them to a paper towel and set aside.

6. Remove the gazpacho from the fridge and divide it between two bowls.
7. Garnish with cilantro and croutons.
8. Serve and enjoy!

Nutrient Breakdown (per one serving):
Calories – 270
Fat in grams – 25
Carbs in grams – 11
Fiber in grams – 2
Protein in grams – 2

# Feta Stuffed Quesadillas (makes 5 servings)

This recipe is where Mexico meets Mediterranean! I love these for the reason that they can be frozen and brought back to life in a pan over low heat. If you're looking to make this recipe even more delicious, look no further than spreading some of the Creamy Dill Sauce as seen in the Dips and Dollops chapter over top of them as well.

Ingredients:
5 whole what tortillas
6 ounces roasted red peppers, sliced
4 ½ ounces black olives, sliced
4 ounces mozzarella cheese, shredded
2 ounces feta cheese, crumbled
½ lb frozen spinach, chopped
½ small red onion
½ teaspoon oregano, minced

Directions:
1. Thaw out the spinach and squeeze out as much moisture as you can with a clean dish towel or paper towel. Transfer the dried spinach to a medium-sized bowl.
2. To this medium-sized bowl, add the roasted red peppers, black olives, red onion, and parsley. Stir until well combined with the spinach.

3. After all ingredients are well combined, add the mozzarella cheese, feta cheese, and oregano. Stir together until all ingredients are evenly distributed.
4. Evenly divide the mixture between your tortillas, spread it out onto only half of the tortilla. Fold the bare side up and overtop the mixture to close it in.
5. Put a pan over medium heat and one-by-one, place your tortillas in, cooking until golden-brown on both sides.
6. Eat, slice, dice, dip, and enjoy!

Nutrient Breakdown (per serving):
Calories – 257
Fat in grams – 12
Carbs in grams – 30
Fiber in grams – 5
Protein in grams – 11

## Collard Leaf Wraps (makes 2 wraps)

Ditch the gluten by wrapping the good stuff in collard leaves! The chickpeas in these mean you'll be full for a while to come, while the abundance of spices means you'll be dreaming about them the day afterwards. The tahini sauce can be found in the Dips and Dollops chapter, and it goes wonderfully with these.

Ingredients:
2 large collard leaves
1 can chickpeas, drained and dried
1 cup quinoa, cooked
½ cup onion, minced
5 artichoke hearts
4 black olives, sliced
4 green olives, sliced
1 red bell pepper, de-seeded and diced
1 garlic clove, minced
3 tablespoons water
3 tablespoons tahini (as seen in the Dips and Dollops chapter)
1 tablespoon olive oil
1 teaspoon lemon juice

¼ teaspoon garlic powder
¼ teaspoon cumin
¼ teaspoon coriander
Dash of pepper
Dash of rosemary

Directions:

1. Preheat oven the 400 degrees Fahrenheit.
2. Prepare a baking sheet by lining it with parchment paper.
3. Put the chickpeas, onion, artichoke hearts, bell pepper, garlic powder, cumin coriander, and rosemary in a medium-sized bowl and give it a gentle toss until well combined.
4. Transfer the mixture to the lined baking sheet and spread it out into an even layer.
5. Place the baking sheet in the oven and let it do its thing for 20 minutes.
6. After 20 minutes, flip the mixture over and bake it for another 7-9 minutes.
7. While the chickpea mixture is in the oven, you can prepare the collard leaves. Do this by bringing a pot of water to a boil and steaming them until tender. Tip: Be sure to de-stem them before you steam them!
8. Once the collard leaves are tender, pat them dry and set them aside for later.
9. Put the tahini, water, lemon juice, garlic, and pepper in a jar and shake ingredients until well combined.
10. By now the chickpea mixture should be done baking and you can begin assembling your wraps. Lay the collard leaves out flat on two separate plates and begin to load them up with all the fixin's. Start by laying the quinoa out in a straight line down the center, then layering the chickpea mixture over top, and finishing with a drizzle of the tahini sauce.
11. Roll the wraps up burrito style. If you're not sure how, check out the diagram in this site:

http://www.mrbreakfast.com/breakfast/wp-content/uploads/2015/03/rolling_frozen_breakfast_burritos.jpg

12. Serve and enjoy!

Nutrient Breakdown (per one wrap):
Calories – 678
Fat in grams – 33
Carbs in grams – 78
Fiber in grams – 17
Protein in grams – 21

# Mediterranean Salad (makes 2 servings)

I imagine this one started as a Greek salad but then too many cooks entered the kitchen, and well – this happened. Regardless, it's fresh, crunchy, delicious, and full of flavor... so I'm really not complaining!

Ingredients:
4 ounces feta cheese, diced
2 cups romaine lettuce, chopped
1 medium tomato, diced
1 medium cucumber, diced
½ small red onion, sliced
Topped with Greek Vinaigrette dressing as seen in the Dips and Dollops chapter

Directions:
1. Add the feta cheese, romaine lettuce, tomato, cucumber, and red onion to a medium-sized bowl. Give this a gentle toss until all ingredients are well combined.
2. Drizzle with the Greek Vinaigrette as seen in the Dips and Dollops chapter and give the salad another toss until all ingredients have a nice coating of the dressing.
3. Divide between two bowls and serve!

Nutrient Breakdown (per one serving):

Calories – 184
Fat in grams – 12
Carbs in grams – 9
Fiber in grams – 3
Protein in grams – 9

## Mediterranean-Style Burger Patties (makes 3 burgers)

These are great alone or wedged between some whole wheat burger buns with fresh toppings. They pair wonderfully with the Potato Skordalia as seen in the Dips and Dollops chapter and are loved amongst children and adults alike. Backyard BBQ, anyone?

Ingredients:
7 ounces chickpeas, rinsed and dried
½ cup old fashioned rolled oats
¼ cup quinoa, cooked
1 small egg
1 garlic clove, minced
2 tablespoons feta cheese, crumbled
2 tablespoons sundried tomatoes, diced
2 tablespoons olive oil
½ tablespoon basil, minced
½ tablespoon parsley, minced
¼ teaspoon oregano
Dash of pepper

Directions:
1. Place your sundried tomatoes in a small bowl and cover them with steaming hot water. Let this stand for 5 minutes or until the tomatoes are rehydrate, then drain and set aside.
2. Put the chickpeas, old fashioned rolled oats, quinoa, garlic, oregano, and pepper into a food processor and pulse until well combined. You'll know it's done when it has the same consistency of hummus. Tip: If your food processor is too small, you can use your blender.

3. Transfer the mixture to a large mixing bowl and add in the feta cheese, sundried tomatoes, basil and parsley. Mix together until all ingredients are thoroughly incorporated.
4. Pick up 1/3 of the mixture and mold it into a round patty. Transfer this to a plate and do the same with the remainder of the mixture.
5. Put a large skillet with the olive oil over medium heat.
6. Once the oil is hot, add in your patties. Cook for 4 minutes on the first side, flip, and then cook for another 4 minutes on the other side. When you're done, both sides should be crispy and golden-brown.
7. Devour and enjoy!

Nutrient Breakdown (per one patty):
Calories – 312
Fat in grams – 18
Carbs in grams – 30
Fiber in grams – 5
Protein in grams – 8

## Portside Tuna Salad (makes about 2 cups)

I love tuna salad for the way it tastes, but also for its affordability and the fact that it is *so* versatile! Dip it, spread it, eat it on its own – you can't go wrong! Plus, the protein will keep you full well into the dinner time hours.

Ingredients:
6 ounces tuna, drained
3 ounces artichoke hearts, drained and diced
3 tablespoons olive oil
2 tablespoons red onion, sliced
2 tablespoons black olives, sliced
½ tablespoon lemon juice
1 teaspoon capers, drained
½ teaspoon oregano
Dash of pepper
Dash of cayenne

Directions:
1.  Add the tuna, artichoke hearts, red onion, black olives, lemon juice, and capers to a bowl. Mix this together until all ingredients are well incorporated.
2.  Drizzle with olive oil and add in your oregano, pepper, and cayenne. Fold this in until the contents have an even coating of oil and spices.
3.  Cover and let sit in the fridge for a half hour or until salad is cold.
4.  Spread, dip, scoop, and enjoy!

Nutrient Breakdown (per ½ cup):
Calories – 142
Fat in grams – 11
Carbs in grams – 3
Fiber in grams – 0
Protein in grams – 9

## Hummus Roll-Ups (makes 6 roll-ups)

Use our Mediterranean-Style Hummus as seen in the Dips and Dollops chapter to really kick the flavor in these up a notch. These are my go-to if I've gone overboard in the morning hours (hey, it happens) or am compensating for some wining and dining later in the day.

Ingredients:
½ large cucumber
3 tablespoons sundried tomatoes, diced
3 tablespoons feta cheese, crumbled
3 tablespoons hummus
Dash of pepper

Directions:
1.  Using a vegetable peeler, peel the dark green skin off your cucumber.
2.  Using the vegetable peeler again, create long, thin ribbons of cucumber.

3. Lay your cucumber ribbons out side-by-side on a clean, flat surface and sprinkle a bit of pepper over each.
4. Spread hummus over your cucumber slices, dividing it evenly as you go.
5. Divide the sundried tomatoes over the hummus.
6. Finish off by crumbling a bit of feta cheese over each cucumber slice.
7. Pick up one end up a cucumber slice and begin to roll it over the hummus. Tip: Roll with caution, as rolling these up too tightly means you'll squish all the filling out.
8. Once the cucumber slice is all rolled up, pierce it with a toothpick to hold it in place.
9. Plate, serve, and enjoy!

Nutrient Breakdown (per one roll-up)
Calories – 32
Fat in grams – 3
Carbs in grams – 3
Fiber in grams – 1
Protein in grams – 3

## Simple Angel Hair Pasta (makes 3 servings)

I love this recipe because it is a perfect balance of simple, savory, and nutritious. The olive oil-rosemary sauce is what really makes this recipe awesome, while the cheeses work to make it creamy and indulgent.

Ingredients:
8 ounces angel hair pasta
¼ cup parmesan cheese, shredded
¼ cup mozzarella cheese, shredded
¼ cup parsley, chopped
¼ cup olive oil
3 garlic cloves, minced
2 tablespoons rosemary, minced
½ teaspoon pepper
¼ teaspoon chili flakes

Directions:
1. Bring a large pot filled with enough water to cover the pasta to a boil.
2. While waiting for the pot to boil, put the olive oil in a saucepan over medium heat.
3. Once the olive oil is hot, add the parsley, garlic, rosemary, and chili flakes, stirring until well combined.
4. Let this mixture sit for one minute or until garlic is fragrant. Then, remove it from the heat and set it aside.
5. Cook the angel hair pasta according to directions on the box and then drain it.
6. Put the pasta back into the pot (but not over heat) and drizzle your seasoned olive oil sauce over top.
7. Finish off by sprinkling the parmesan cheese, mozzarella cheese, and pepper overtop or stirring it in. This part is up to you!
8. Divide the pasta between two bowls, serve with a side of whole wheat toast, and enjoy!

Nutrient Breakdown (per one serving):
Calories – 487
Fat in grams – 23
Carbs in grams – 59
Fiber in grams – 3
Protein in grams – 15

# Chapter 6 – Dinner for Winners

## Baked Sweet Potatoes with Crunchy Chickpeas (makes 2 servings)

It's a classic with a delicious Mediterranean twist! Baked chickpeas do a lovely job of complimenting the sweet potato, while the hummus completes the meal in a way which is both savory and nutritious.

Ingredients:
4 medium sweet potatoes, cleaned and halved
1 can chickpeas, rinsed and dried
¼ cup hummus
3 garlic cloves, minced
1 tablespoon lemon juice
1 tablespoon water
1 tablespoon olive oil
1 teaspoon dill
Dash of coriander
Dash of paprika
Dash of cinnamon
Dash of cumin

Directions:
1. Preheat oven to 400 degrees Fahrenheit.
2. Prepare a baking sheet by lining it with parchment paper.
3. In a bowl, mix together the chickpeas, half the olive oil, coriander, paprika, cinnamon, and cumin.
4. Transfer this mixture to the baking sheet, spreading it out over half the sheet in an even layer.
5. Rub the open halves of the sweet potatoes with the remaining olive oil. Then, transfer them to the free space reserved on the baking sheet.
6. Place the baking sheet in the oven and let bake for 45 minutes or until sweet potatoes are tender. Tip: Make

sure to periodically rotate the chickpeas to ensure they don't burn.

7. While the baking sheet is in the oven, stir the hummus, garlic, lemon juice, water, and dill together in a small bowl until well combined.
8. Once the chickpeas have a golden-brown color and the sweet potatoes are tender, remove them from the oven.
9. Let the potatoes cool until you can touch them and then divide them between two plates.
10. Spread the hummus mixture over them, dividing it evenly as you go.
11. Sprinkle the crunchy chickpeas over top.
12. Serve and enjoy!

Nutrient Breakdown (per one serving):
Calories – 699
Fat in grams – 25
Carbs in grams – 102
Fiber in grams – 22
Protein in grams – 20

# Oven Baked Cauliflower (makes 1 serving)

This one is perfect for those busy nights when cooking really isn't a first priority. It's nutritious yet as simple as throwing the ingredients together and letting the oven do the rest. Not to mention, it's mouth-wateringly creamy thanks to the melted parmesan cheese.

Ingredients:
1 small cauliflower, broken into florets
3 garlic cloves, minced
1 tablespoon parmesan cheese
1 tablespoon lemon juice
¼ teaspoon pepper
Chives to garnish

Directions:
1. Preheat oven to 500 degrees Fahrenheit.

2. Put your cauliflower florets into a medium-sized roasting pan.
3. Pour the olive oil and lemon juice over the florets.
4. Sprinkle the garlic and pepper over the florets.
5. Place the roasting pan in the oven and let bake for 10 minutes or until florets are tender, stirring every once in a while.
6. Remove the roasting pan from the oven and finish off by sprinkling the parmesan cheese and chives overtop.
7. Dish out, serve with a side of your choice, and enjoy!

Nutrient Breakdown (per one serving):
Calories – 102
Fat in grams – 1
Carbs in grams – 18
Fiber in grams – 7
Protein in grams – 8

# Zesty Lime Baked Chicken (makes 3 servings)

I love doubling this recipe to bring to a potluck or serve to hungry guests in my own home. The chicken always comes up wonderfully crispy while the cilantro, lime juice, and spices help to bring out some unexpected, refreshing flavor. Serve with the Tzatziki as seen in the Dips and Dollops chapter and the meal is complete!

Ingredients:
4 chicken thighs
1 cup chicken broth
½ cup white wine (dry is best)
¼ cup cilantro, de-stemmed and chopped
3 garlic cloves, chopped
2 tablespoons lime juice
2 tablespoons olive oil
½ tablespoon garlic powder
½ teaspoon pepper
½ teaspoon paprika
¼ teaspoon nutmeg

Directions:

1. Preheat oven to 375 degrees Fahrenheit.
2. In a small bowl, stir together the garlic powder, pepper, paprika, and nutmeg until well combined.
3. Rub this spice mixture into the chicken thighs, dividing it evenly as you go.
4. After you're done spicing the chicken, let them sit to marinate for about 20 minutes.
5. Put a skillet with the olive oil over medium-high heat.
6. Once the oil is hot, add in the chicken and let it brown on both sides.
7. Once the chicken is nicely browned, transfer it to a plate and set aside.
8. Lower the heat and pour in the white wine.
9. Once most of the white wine evaporates, add in the broth. Let this mixture come to a simmer.
10. Once you've reached a simmer, add in the garlic and lime juice.
11. Once the garlic become fragrant, add the chicken back in, this time adding the cilantro with it.
12. Up the heat a little and let this come to a very active simmer for about 3 minutes.
13. Cover the skillet with its corresponding lid and transfer it to the oven. Let the chicken bake for 30 minutes or until cooked through.
14. Remove the skillet from the oven and let it cool for a couple minutes before serving.
15. Plate, serve with a side of colorful veggies, and enjoy!

Nutrient Breakdown (per one serving):
Calories – 309
Fat in grams – 22
Carbs in grams – 2
Fiber in grams – 0
Protein in grams – 21

## Savory Kale Spaghetti (makes 2 servings)

If you have trouble getting your kids to eat their veggies, this dish may be your answer. It has a colossal amount of kale full of nutrients and antioxidants that's overpowered by the deliciousness of feta cheese, garlic, and cherry tomatoes. Here's to a dinner time classic turned Mediterranean – now it's more nutritious than ever thought possible!

Ingredients:
½ package whole wheat spaghetti noodles
3-4 cups kale leaves (packed), de-stemmed and chopped
¼ cup feta cheese, crumbled
15 cherry tomatoes, halved
2 garlic cloves, minced
2 ½ tablespoons olive oil
Dash of pepper

Directions:
1. Put a saucepan with half of the olive oil over medium heat.
2. Once the oil is hot, add the kale leaves and let cook until wilted.
3. Once the kale leaves are wilted, add the cherry tomatoes, garlic, and pepper and cook until fragrant. Then, stir in the remaining olive oil, remove it from heat, and set it aside.
4. Bring a pot with enough water to cover the spaghetti noodles to a boil.
5. Once boiling, add the spaghetti noodles and cook them according to the directions on the box.
6. Once the spaghetti noodles are cooked to your preference, drain off the water and put them back in the pot.
7. Pour the contents of the saucepan into the pot.
8. Toss the spaghetti noodles with the olive oil sauce until all noodles have an even coating of it.
9. Finish by stirring in the feta cheese.
10. Divide into two bowls, serve with some olives on the side, and enjoy!

Nutrient Breakdown (per one serving):
Calories – 407
Fat in grams – 23
Carbs in grams – 41
Fiber in grams – 2
Protein in grams – 12

## Shrimp on a Stick (makes 1 serving)

Who doesn't love a good shrimp kebab every now and then? The simple marinade included with this recipe compliments the shrimp and artichokes beautifully, but if you're looking to up your sauce game a bit the Spicy Cilantro Sauce as seen in the Dips and Dollops is absolutely magnificent as well.

Kebab Ingredients:
170 grams large shrimp, deveined and shelled
6 small artichoke hearts
6 black olives, pitted
2 tablespoons feta cheese, crumbled

Marinade Ingredients:
2 tablespoons lemon juice
2 tablespoons olive oil
1 teaspoon lemon zest
½ teaspoon Italian seasoning

Directions:
1. Put the lemon juice, olive oil, lemon zest, and Italian seasoning in a freezer bag, seal it, and squish the ingredients together until well combined.
2. Add the shrimp to the bag and shake it up until each has a nice coating of the marinade.
3. Place freezer bag with shrimp in the fridge and let the flavors soak through overnight, giving it a good shake every once in a while. Tip: If you're crunched for time, 4 hours of marinating will be sufficient.
4. Once the shrimp is marinated to your liking, you can begin to prepare the rest of the kebab ingredients. Add

the artichoke hearts and black olives to the freezer bag and shake it around until they have a nice, even coating of the marinade.

5.  Thread shrimp, artichoke hearts, and olives onto 2 kebab skewers. Be as creative and varied as you wish.
6.  Heat a grill to medium direct heat.
7.  Once the grill is ready, place the skewers on it and let them cook, covered, for 5-8 minutes. Turn these once or twice while they cook to ensure they cook evenly.
8.  Once the shrimp is cooked through, transfer the skewers to a plate and finish off with a sprinkle of the feta cheese.
9.  Serve and enjoy!

Nutrient Breakdown (per one serving):
Calories – 500
Fat in grams – 34
Carbs in grams – 8
Fiber in grams – 2
Protein in grams – 36

## Tomato Layered Fish (makes 2 servings)

Think crispy, breaded fish with a refreshing salsa-like sauce over top. If you're low on protein by the end of the day this dish is a great way to up it, not to mention delicious along with a glass of red wine.

Ingredients:
½ lb fish filets (of your choice)
½ can chopped tomatoes
¼ cup whole wheat bread crumbs
1 medium onion, minced
½ carrot, chopped
½ celery stalk, chopped
1 garlic clove, minced
2 tablespoons olive oil
1 tablespoon parsley, minced
½ tablespoon lemon juice

½ tablespoon tomato paste
¼ teaspoon sugar
¼ teaspoon oregano

Directions:
1. Preheat oven to 350 degrees Fahrenheit.
2. Put a frying pan with half the olive oil over medium heat.
3. Once the oil is hot, add the onion, carrot, and celery. Let this cook until soft and tender.
4. Once the onion, carrot, and celery are soft and tender, add the garlic and cook for 2 minutes or until fragrant.
5. Once the garlic is fragrant, reduce the heat to low and add the chopped tomatoes, parsley, lemon juice, tomato paste, sugar, and oregano. Let this simmer for 10 minutes or until it becomes a thick sauce.
6. While your veggies simmer, place the fish filets on a lined baking dish side-by-side.
7. Once your sauce is ready, evenly distribute it over the fish filets and drizzle the remaining olive oil over top.
8. Place the baking dish in the oven and let it bake for 15-20 minutes, or until your fish is flaky and cooked through.
9. Plate, serve, and enjoy!

Nutrient Breakdown (per one serving):
Calories – 310
Fat in grams – 16
Carbs in grams – 20
Fiber in grams – 5
Protein in grams – 20

## Tomato Eggplant Bake (makes 2 servings)

The veggies in this meal are paired with a beautiful array of spices which bring out their flavors. It's a great way to get all your servings of veggies in one shot if you're still lacking in that department come night time. This dish can also be transformed into something completely different by adding some whole wheat noodles or a bit of brown rice.

Ingredients:
2 baby eggplants, halved with ends discarded
¼ cup water
1 medium red onion, sliced
1 medium tomato, diced
2-3 fresh mint leaves
2 garlic cloves, minced
2 ½ tablespoons olive oil
2 tablespoons roasted almonds, chopped
1 ½ tablespoons tomato paste
1/8 teaspoon cumin
1/8 teaspoon paprika
Dash of pepper

Directions:
1. Preheat oven to 375 degrees Fahrenheit.
2. Put the eggplant and olive oil in a medium-sized bowl and toss gently until eggplant has a nice coating of the oil.
3. Transfer the eggplant to a lined baking sheet with the cut side face-down.
4. Put the baking sheet in the oven and bake for 15-20 minutes or until the eggplant begins to turn golden-brown. Tip: Flip them halfway through for a more even bake.
5. While the eggplant bakes, put a pan with 1 ½ tablespoons olive oil over medium-high heat.
6. Once the oil is hot, add the onion and cook for 5 minutes or until it is translucent.
7. Once the onion is translucent, add the garlic and cook for 1 minute or until fragrant.
8. Once the garlic is fragrant, add the tomato, cumin, paprika, and pepper. Cook this for 3-5 minutes or until the tomatoes begin to break down.
9. Once the tomatoes have broken down a bit, add in the water and tomato pasta and let cook for 5 minutes or

until the sauce thickens up. Then, remove the pan from heat.
10. By now your eggplant should be done. Remove it from the oven and divide the pieces between two plates.
11. Pour your tomato sauce over top and garnish with the toasted almonds and fresh mint.
12. Serve warm and enjoy!

Nutrient Breakdown (per one serving):
Calories – 374
Fat in grams – 24
Carbs in grams – 40
Fiber in grams – 20
Protein in grams – 9

# Tomato Patties (makes 4 patties)

This makes for quite the unorthodox meal, but it's delicious nonetheless. Pair it with the creamy dill sauce as seen in the Dips and Dollops to create a meal that's truly unforgettable.

Ingredients:
1 large tomato, chopped
¼ red onion, minced
2 tablespoons olive oil
½ tablespoon mint, minced
1 teaspoon parsley, minced
Dash of pepper

Directions:
1. Put the whole wheat flour, tomato, red onion, mint, parsley, and 1 teaspoon olive oil in a medium-sized bowl. Fold ingredients in until well combined. Tip: When you're done, the mixture should look like a thick batter.
2. Cover the bowl with plastic wrap and let the mixture sit for 20 minutes.
3. After the mixture has sat for 20 minutes, put a pan with the remaining olive oil over medium heat.

4. Once the oil is hot, scoop the mixture into the pan, creating 4 "patties" in total.
5. Let the patties cook for 2-3 minutes each side or until golden-brown all around.
6. Plate 2 patties on each plate, serve between whole wheat burger buns or with a side of veggies, and enjoy!

Nutrient Breakdown (per one patty):
Calories – 68
Fat in grams – 7
Carbs in grams – 3
Fiber in grams – 1
Protein in grams – 1

# Spicy Quinoa and Chickpea Salad (makes 4 servings)

This salad is full of protein and a healthy balance of other nutrients to keep you full and satisfied until the next morning. If spice isn't really your thing, simply remove the jalapenos from the dressing – it's still refreshing and delicious without them!

Salad Ingredients:
1 medium cauliflower, divided into florets
3 cups chickpeas, drained and rinsed
2 cups quinoa, cooked and cooled
½ cup roasted almonds, chopped
¼ cup mint leaves, torn
¼ cup parsley leaves, chopped
¼ cup cilantro leaves, chopped
3 tablespoons olive oil
2 tablespoons lemon zest
2 teaspoons cumin seeds

Dressing Ingredients:
3 jalapenos, minced
¼ cup chives, chopped
¼ cup lime juice

¼ cup olive oil
Dash of pepper

Directions:
1. Preheat oven to 430 degrees Fahrenheit.
2. Put the cauliflower florets, ½ the lemon zest, ½ the olive oil, and pepper in a medium-sized bowl. Give the ingredients a good toss until cauliflower florets are nicely coated in seasonings.
3. Transfer the seasoned cauliflower florets to a lined baking sheet.
4. Place the baking sheet in the oven and let bake for 20-25 minutes or until cauliflower is gold and tender. Tip: Rotate the florets every 5 minutes to ensure they bake evenly.
5. While the cauliflower florets are in the oven, put the chickpeas, remaining lemon zest, remaining olive oil, cumin seeds, and pepper in another medium-sized bowl. Give these ingredients a good toss until the chickpeas are also coated in seasonings.
6. Transfer the chickpeas to another lined baking sheet and spread them out into an even layer.
7. Once the cauliflower florets are done, remove them from the oven and put the chickpeas in. Roast the chickpeas for 20-25 minutes or until they are crispy and golden-brown. Tip: Rotate the chickpeas every 5 minutes to ensure they bake evenly.
8. While the chickpeas are in the oven, put the jalapeno, chives, lime juice, olive oil, and pepper in a jar and give it a good shake.
9. Remove the chickpeas from the oven.
10. Allow cauliflower and chickpeas to cool. Tip: You can speed up this process using the fridge, freezer, or even the great outdoors if it's cold enough!
11. Once the cauliflower and chickpeas are cool, transfer them into a large-sized mixing bowl.
12. To the large-sized mixing bowl, add the quinoa, roasted almonds, mint leaves, parsley leaves, and cilantro leaves.

13. Drizzle the dressing over top and give the salad a gentle toss until all ingredients have an even coating.
14. Divide salad between four bowls, serve with a glass of wine, and enjoy!

Nutrient Breakdown (per one serving):
Calories – 597
Fat in grams – 35
Carbs in grams – 60
Fiber in grams – 17
Protein in grams – 19

# Gluten-Free Zucchini Pizza (makes 4 servings)

This pizza is a great way to ensure you get all your servings of veggies! The eggplant dough is a little unorthodox, but crispy and chewy nonetheless. Serve with some Lemon Caper Sauce as seen in the Dips and Dollops chapter to finish this number off!

Ingredients:
4 Italian eggplants
¾ cup ground flaxseed
½ cup almond flour
½ cup feta cheese, crumbled
1 graffiti eggplant, sliced thin
1 baby eggplant, sliced thin
1 green zucchini, sliced thin
1 yellow zucchini, sliced thin
2 eggs
1 tomato, sliced thin
2 tablespoons + 2 teaspoons olive oil
½ teaspoon pepper

Directions:
1. Peel the Italian eggplants.
2. Shred the Italian eggplants using a cheese grated. Set aside for 10 minutes.

3. Squeeze all excess moisture out of the eggplants with the clean dish towel, paper towels, or cheesecloth.
4. Preheat oven to 375 degrees Fahrenheit.
5. Transfer the shredded eggplant to a large-sized mixing bowl and fold in the ground flaxseed, almond flour, eggs, 2 tablespoons olive oil, and pepper until a dough-like substance forms.
6. Mold the dough into a ball and transfer it to a lined baking sheet.
7. Press dough out into an even layer about ¼ inch thick. Tip: This recipe makes a lot of pizza, so you may have to work in batches.
8. Place baking sheet on the oven's middle rack and let bake for 20 minutes.
9. After 20 minutes, remove the baking sheet from the oven and lay another piece of parchment paper over top the dough.
10. Place another baking sheet over top (face down), and flip so that the dough transfers to the baking sheet on top.
11. Peel off what used to be the bottom layer of parchment paper and discard of it.
12. Brush the pizza crust with remaining olive oil.
13. Evenly distribute the graffiti eggplant, baby eggplant, green zucchini, yellow zucchini, and tomato over the pizza crust.
14. Sprinkle feta cheese over top.
15. Place pizza back in the oven, this time baking it for 15-20 minutes or until the corners of the crust are golden-brown and crispy.
16. Slice, serve, and enjoy!

Nutrient Breakdown (per one serving):
Calories – 561
Fat in grams – 31
Carbs in grams – 62
Fiber in grams – 39
Protein in grams –24

# Roasted Tomato Bowls (makes 4 bowls)

When you've got friends coming over to enjoy the evening, these tomato bowls are sure to be a hit! While they may not look like much, they're filled to the brim (literally) with nutritious ingredients to keep you full and keep the conversation going!

Ingredients:
4 large tomatoes
2 cups mushrooms, diced
½ cup pearl barley
¼ cup parmesan cheese, shredded
¼ cup + 1 tablespoon olive oil
1 egg
½ zucchini, diced
1 tablespoon Italian seasoning
Dash of pepper

Directions:
1. Preheat oven to 375 degrees Fahrenheit.
2. Slice the tops off of your tomatoes and set them aside for later.
3. With a spoon, carefully scoop out the insides of the tomatoes and transfer them to a bowl.
4. Mash the tomato insides with a potato masher or fork until liquid-y. Set this aside.
5. Turn the tomatoes upside down over a paper towel to drain off the excess juice.
6. While the tomatoes "drain" themselves, put a large frying pan with ¼ cup oil over medium-high heat.
7. Once the oil is hot, add the mushrooms, zucchini, and Italian seasoning. Let this cook until the zucchini is tender.
8. Once the zucchini is tender, pour in the mashed-up tomato insides and pearl barley. Stir until all ingredients are well combined.

9. Once all ingredients are well combined, crack the egg and dump the parmesan into it as well. Give this another good stir and then remove the pan from heat.
10. Fill the tomatoes with the frying pan mixture, dividing it evenly as you go. Tip: Be sure to pack the frying pan mixture into the tomatoes tightly with a spoon or spatula.
11. Once the tomatoes are stuffed, place them on a lined baking sheet and put their lids back on.
12. Drizzle the remaining olive oil over the tomatoes and place them in the oven for 35-40 minutes or until the filling is hot and the tomatoes appear to be wilted.
13. Place two tomato bowls on one plate, two tomato bowls on another, pour yourself a glass of wine, and enjoy!

Nutrient Breakdown (per 1 tomato bowl):
Calories – 303
Fat in grams – 20
Carbs in grams – 27
Fiber in grams – 7
Protein in grams – 8

## Savory & Spicy Shrimp Spaghetti (makes 2 servings)

When you need to add some protein to your day, look no further than this beautiful Mediterranean-style spaghetti. The sauce is what makes this dish – incorporating all factors of spicy, creamy, and nutritious.

Ingredients:
110 grams whole wheat spaghetti
12 jumbo shrimp, cleaned and steamed
2 cups chopped tomatoes
¼ cup yoghurt, low-fat
2 garlic cloves, minced
2 anchovy filets, chopped
2 tablespoons basil, minced
1 ½ tablespoons olive oil

1 tablespoon balsamic vinegar
1 tablespoon capers, drained
½ tablespoon brown sugar
½ teaspoon cayenne
¼ teaspoon chili flakes
Dash of pepper

Directions:
1. Put the yoghurt in a coffee filter lined strainer and let this sit in the fridge for an hour or until most liquid drains. Tip: Be sure to put this contraption over a bowl or container to catch the liquid!
2. Once your yoghurt is ready, put a pan with the olive oil over medium heat.
3. Once the oil is hot, add the garlic and let cook for about 1 minute or until fragrant.
4. Once garlic is fragrant, add the tomatoes, anchovies, balsamic vinegar, capers, brown sugar, and pepper. Let this cook until the sauce starts to thicken.
5. Once the sauce is thick, stir in the shrimp, yoghurt, basil, cayenne, and chili flakes until all ingredients are well combined. Remove from heat and set aside.
6. Cook spaghetti according to directions on the package.
7. Once spaghetti is cooked to your preference, drain the water and put it back into the pot.
8. Pour the sauce into the spaghetti pot and toss until spaghetti has a nice, even coating of the sauce.
9. Divide between two bowls, serve with some veggies on the side, and enjoy!

Nutrient Breakdown (per one serving):
Calories – 480
Fat in grams – 15
Carbs in grams – 54
Fiber in grams – 8
Protein in grams – 34

# Tomato Basil Stuffed Peppers (makes 4 peppers)

Think tacos, but with a crunchy bell pepper shell instead. I like to get creative with these and experiment with different fillings. This recipe, however, is my original and has yet to be beat!

Ingredients:
1 lb chicken, ground
4 bell peppers of your color preference
1 can of tomato sauce
1 ½ cups brown rice, cooked
1/3 cup heavy cream
¼ cup basil, chopped
¾ cup feta cheese
3 garlic cloves, minced
½ onion, diced
1 tablespoon olive oil
Dash of pepper

Directions:
1. Preheat oven to 400 degrees Fahrenheit.
2. Slice the tops of the peppers off and scoop out their insides. Discard of them and set the peppers aside.
3. Put the chicken in a bowl and fold the pepper into it until evenly distributed.
4. Put a pan with the olive oil over medium heat.
5. Once the oil is hot, add the onion and let it cook for about 5 minutes or until translucent.
6. Once the onion is translucent, add 2 garlic cloves and cook for 1 minute or until fragrant.
7. Once the garlic is fragrant, add the seasoned ground chicken and let it cook for 10-15 minutes or until cooked through.
8. While the chicken cooks, mix the tomato sauce with the heavy cream and remaining garlic clove.
9. Transfer this mixture to a saucepan over low heat and stir in some basil, leaving a little bit to garnish your peppers later.

10. Stir the brown rice and feta cheese into the chicken mixture until well combined.
11. Once well combined, pour half of the tomato sauce mixture into the pan and stir again until well combined. Remove from heat.
12. Line your bell peppers up nearby and divide the frying pan mixture between them, pouring it into each pepper until full.
13. Spoon about 2 teaspoons of the remaining cream sauce into each pepper.
14. Transfer the peppers to a baking pan and pour the remainder of the tomato sauce into the bottom of the pan.
15. Place the tops back on the peppers and stick them in the oven for 20 minutes.
16. Remove the baking pan from the oven and cover the peppers with aluminum foil.
17. Place the baking pan back in the oven and cook for an additional 30 minutes.
18. Remove the baking pan from the oven, discard of the aluminum foil, and garnish with the remaining basil.
19. Place 2 peppers on each plate, serve with a glass of wine, and enjoy!

Nutrient Breakdown (per 1 pepper):
Calories – 559
Fat in grams – 29
Carbs in grams – 34
Fiber in grams – 6
Protein in grams – 39

# Veggie and Rice Casserole (makes 2 servings)

This one is a Mediterranean classic with the American spin of comforting casserole! If you wish, you can double this recipe and freeze parts of it for those nights when you really just don't feel like cooking.

Ingredients:

1 cup brown rice, cooked
¼ cup parsley, chopped
¼ cup spinach, chopped
1 medium onion, chopped
2 garlic cloves, minced
2 tablespoons roasted almonds, sliced
2 tablespoons olive oil
1 ½ tablespoons lemon juice
1 tablespoon balsamic vinegar
½ tablespoon dill weed
1 teaspoon thyme
½ teaspoon allspice
¼ teaspoon paprika
¼ teaspoon cinnamon
Dash of pepper

Directions:
1. Preheat oven to 350 degrees Fahrenheit.
2. Put a pot with the olive oil over medium-high heat.
3. Once the oil is hot, add the onion and garlic and cook for about 10 minutes or until the onion begins to brown.
4. Once the onions begin to brown, add in the parsley, spinach, roasted almonds, lemon juice, balsamic vinegar, dill weed, thyme, allspice, paprika, cinnamon, and pepper. Stir all ingredients together until well combined.
5. Turn heat down to medium, put a lid over the pot, and allow mixture to simmer for about 5 minutes or until the greens begin to wilt.
6. Dump in the brown rice and fold into the rest of the ingredients until well incorporated. Then, remove the pot from the heat.
7. Spray down a casserole dish with some cooking spray and transfer the brown rice mixture into it.
8. Place the baking dish in the oven and bake for 20 minutes or until heated through.
9. Divide dish between two plates, serve with some veggies on the side, and enjoy!

Nutrient Breakdown (per one serving):
Calories – 334
Fat in grams – 22
Carbs in grams – 30
Fiber in grams – 5
Protein in grams – 7

## Onion Fried Eggs (makes two servings)

This dish is incredibly easy to throw together yet oh-so delicious. Made with budget-friendly foods you can find at your nearest grocery store, you can serve the whole family an awesome, nutritious meal without going broke!

Ingredients:
8 eggs
85 grams feta cheese, crumbled
1/3 cup (packed) sundried tomatoes, chopped
1 large onion, sliced
1 garlic clove, minced
2 tablespoons olive oil
Dash of pepper

Directions:
1. Put a pan with the olive oil over medium-low heat.
2. Once the oil is hot, add the onions and stir them into the oil.
3. Allow the onions to cook for about one hour, or until they become a deep brown color. Tip: Stir them every 5-7 minutes to ensure they cook evenly.
4. After the onions have browned, add the sundried tomatoes and garlic and let cook for 2 minutes or until fragrant.
5. Once the sundried tomatoes and garlic are fragrant, spread all the ingredients out into an even, thin layer across the pan.
6. Crack the eggs overtop the ingredients already in the pan.

7. Sprinkle your feta cheese and pepper over top of the eggs.
8. Cover the pan with its corresponding lid and let the eggs sit to cook for about 10-12 minutes. Tip: Gently shake the pan at 10 minutes to check on the consistency of the egg yolks. Continue to cook until they reach your desired level of doneness.
9. Remove pan from heat and divide the mixture between two plates.
10. Serve, maybe with some whole wheat bread on the side, and enjoy!

Nutrient Breakdown (per one serving):
Calories – 661
Fat in grams – 43
Carbs in grams – 21
Fiber in grams – 7
Protein in grams – 35

# Chapter 7 – Sides n' Snacks

## Crispy Falafel (makes 12 patties)

While these patties are great on their own, they're best known for being stuffed into pitas and served over salads. The bright green color of these is especially staggering, not that the spices aren't enough to make them something to remember.

Ingredients:
1 cup chickpeas, drained and rinsed
½ cup parsley, chopped with stems removed
1/3 cup cilantro, chopped with stems removed
¼ cup dill, chopped with stems removed
4 garlic cloves, minced
1 tablespoon sesame seeds, toasted
½ tablespoon coriander
½ tablespoon black pepper
½ tablespoon cumin
½ teaspoon baking powder
½ teaspoon cayenne
Olive oil for frying

Directions:
1. Thoroughly dry your chickpeas with a paper towel.
2. Place the parsley, cilantro, and dill in a food processor and pulse until it forms mulch.
3. Once mulch has formed, add in the chickpeas, garlic, coriander, black pepper, cumin, baking powder, and cayenne. Pulse this mixture until smooth and well combined.
4. Transfer the mixture to an air tight container and let it sit in the fridge for about an hour, or until stiff.
5. Remove the mixture from the fridge and stir in the baking powder and sesame seeds until well combined.
6. Scoop the mixture into a pan with 3 inches of olive oil over medium heat to create patties. Keep in mind as

you create the patties that you're aiming to make 12 with the mixture.

7. Let the falafel patties fry for 1-2 minutes on each side or until golden-brown.
8. Once your falafel patties are nicely browned, transfer them to a plate lined with paper towels to finish crisping.
9. Dip, dunk, fill, and enjoy!

Nutrient Breakdown (per one patty):
Calories – 102
Fat in grams – 5
Carbs in grams – 12
Fiber in grams – 3
Protein in grams – 4

## Pita Crisps (makes 48 crisps)

Pair these with the Mediterranean-Style Hummus as seen in the Dips and Dollops recipe to create a traditional Mediterranean snack! While these are simple and require little effort to make, they're absolutely delightful. I'm sure you'll be making them over and over again!

Ingredients:
6 whole wheat pitas
1/3 cup olive oil
1 teaspoon garlic powder
1 teaspoon black pepper

Directions:
1. Preheat oven to 375 degrees Fahrenheit.
2. Brush both sides of each pita with a generous amount of the olive oil.
3. Using a pizza cutter, slice each pita 4 times to create 8 even wedges
4. Toss these wedges in a bowl with the garlic powder and salt until they have an even coating of spices.

5.   Place the pita wedges on a lined baking sheet and bake them in the oven for 15-17 minutes or until crispy.
6.   Let cool, serve with some dip, and enjoy!

Nutrient Breakdown (per ten crisps):
Calories – 336
Fat in grams – 16
Carbs in grams – 45
Fiber in grams – 6
Protein in grams – 8

# Zucchini Discs (makes 4 discs)

Soft on the outside and crispy on the inside, these are sure to be a favorite in the household. I love pairing mine with some of the Traditional Mediterranean Aioli as seen in the Dips and Dollops chapter, but they are great on their own too!

Ingredients:
2 zucchinis
1 cup whole wheat flour
¼ cup parsley, chopped
¼ cup dill, chopped
2 small eggs
1 scallion
2 tablespoons mint
2 tablespoons chives
½ tablespoon paprika
½ teaspoon pepper
Olive oil for frying

Directions:
1.   Peel and grate your zucchini.
2.   Once you've grated the zucchini, wring out all the excess water using cheesecloth, clean dish cloth, or paper towels.
3.   Once all the excess liquid has been removed, place the zucchini in a colander to finish draining for 10 minutes.

4. Grate the carrot while you wait for the zucchini to finish draining.
5. Place the eggs in a bowl with the paprika and pepper. Whisk together until well combined.
6. In a large mixing bowl, mix together the zucchini, carrot, feta cheese, and egg mixture until well combined.
7. Sift in the flour as you mix and keep mixing until a dough-like substance forms.
8. Put a pan with the olive oil over medium heat.
9. Once the oil is hot, use a spoon to drop the zucchini mixture into it.
10. Fry your zucchini patties for a couple minutes on each side, or until golden brown.
11. Once your patties are golden brown, place them on a surface lined with paper towel to finish crisping.
12. Serve and enjoy!

Nutrient Breakdown (per one disc):
Calories – 255
Fat in grams – 13
Carbs in grams – 31
Fiber in grams – 3
Protein in grams – 8

## Spicy Potato Chunks (makes 4 servings)

When asked what my favorite food is, I never hesitate. Potatoes, 100%. They taste great baked, mashed, as fries, as hash browns... I could go on forever. This recipe in particular creates a side which is nicely spiced, crunchy, and surprisingly refreshing. Not to mention, getting them made up is a snap.

Ingredients:
5 russet potatoes
2 ½ tablespoons olive oil
2 garlic cloves, minced
2 tablespoons cilantro, minced
½ teaspoon paprika

½ teaspoon cumin
½ teaspoon coriander
½ teaspoon pepper
1 teaspoon cayenne pepper

Directions:
1. Preheat oven to 450 degrees Fahrenheit.
2. Peel the potatoes and cut them into bite-sized chunks.
3. Transfer the potato chunks to a bowl and drizzle with 1 ½ tablespoons of the olive oil. Gently toss the potatoes in the olive oil until they are nicely coated.
4. Spread the potato chunks across a baking sheet lined with parchment paper and bake in the oven for 35-40 minutes or until they are crispy and have a beautiful golden color.
5. Once the potatoes are nicely baked, remove them from the oven and transfer them to a medium-sized bowl. Set aside.
6. In a saucepan, mix the remaining oil with the garlic until well combined.
7. Place this saucepan over medium heat and let it cook for one minute or until fragrant.
8. Add the paprika, cumin, coriander, pepper, and cayenne pepper to the sauce pan and stir until well combined.
9. Once the spices have been over heat for about 2 minutes, use a spatula to drizzle the oil seasoning over your potatoes. Make sure you get every last drop! The stuff is delicious.
10. Toss the potatoes with the oil seasoning until they are nicely coated.
11. Lastly, add in the cilantro and give the potatoes one last toss.
12. Serve and enjoy!

Nutrient Breakdown (per one serving):
Calories – 265
Fat in grams – 9
Carbs in grams – 43

Fiber in grams – 7
Protein in grams – 5

## Traditional Dolmades (makes 10 dolmades)

A dolmade is a traditional Greek roll made up of grape leaves and a rice filling. This rice filling in particular is tangy with a wonderful flavor of onion. Bring them to a party to impress your friends or, like I do, eat the entire platter yourself on a Saturday night in the company of your cats. The choice is yours!

Ingredients:
10 grape leaves in brine, drained
½ small onion
½ green onion, minced
2 ½ tablespoons round grain rice
2 ½ tablespoons olive oil
½ tablespoon lemon juice
½ tablespoon long grain rice
½ tablespoon dill, minced
1 teaspoon parsley, minced
Dash of mint, minced

Directions:
1. Heat 1 1/3 tablespoons olive oil in a pan over medium-high heat.
2. Once the oil is hot, add in your onions and cook for ½ minute or until fragrant.
3. Once onions are fragrant, add in your rice and ½ cup of water.
4. Bring this mixture to a boil and cook for another minute afterwards.
5. Stir in the dill, parsley, and mint until well combined. Then, remove from heat and set aside.
6. Drizzle the remaining olive oil into the bottom of a small pot and tilt until the bottom has a nice, even coating of it.
7. Lay out your grape vine leaves vein side up.

8. Spoon the rice mixture onto the center of the leaves, dividing evenly as you go.
9. Once all the leaves have a spoonful of the rice mixture, roll them up burrito-style. If you're not sure what I'm talking about, check out the diagram in this site: http://www.mrbreakfast.com/breakfast/wp-content/uploads/2015/03/rolling_frozen_breakfast_b urritos.jpg
10. Transfer the rolled dolmades, seam side down, to the oil-coated pot. Put the pot over medium-high heat.
11. Once all of the dolmades are in the pot, drizzle with a splash of olive oil and enough water to cover them.
12. Place a plate over the dolmades to weigh them down and bring the pot to a boil.
13. Once the pot is boiling, reduce the heat to medium-low and simmer for 10-20 minutes, or until the rice is tender.
14. Serve and enjoy!

Nutrient Breakdown (per one dolmade):
Calories – 40
Fat in grams – 4
Carbs in grams – 2
Fiber in grams – 0
Protein in grams – 0

# Chapter 8 – Dips & Dollops

## Simple Tahini (makes 2 cups)

This traditional Middle-Eastern sauce is made with a base of sesame seeds along with other seasonings. Some of the dishes in this book call for a splash of it, including some sauces in this chapter. It is for this reason I decided to keep it super simple. It's still delicious, just without all the complexity.

Ingredients:
2 cups sesame seeds
¼ cup olive oil
1 teaspoon sesame oil

Directions:
1. Place a skillet with the sesame seeds over medium heat, stirring them slowly with a wooden spoon.
2. Let the seeds toast for about 5 minutes or until fragrant. Tip: Do *not* toast them so long that they begin to brown.
3. Transfer the seeds to a baking sheet and spread them out in an even layer. Let them cool like this.
4. Once the sesame seeds have cooled, transfer them to a food processor and pulse until they turn into a crumbly paste.
5. Once the sesame seeds have turned into a crumbly paste, add the oils and process again, this time until the mixture is thick yet fairly smooth.
6. Store in a jar or air tight container and use as needed! Give the tahini a good stir before each use.

Nutrient Breakdown (per one tablespoon):
Calories – 69
Fat in grams – 6
Carbs in grams – 2
Fiber in grams – 2
Protein in grams – 2

# Mediterranean-Style Hummus (makes 3 cups)

While hummus alone comes from the Mediterranean region, this version gives it an especially Greek twist. If you want to simplify it to the traditional hummus, you can do so easily by eliminating the crushed red pepper and cumin. It's that easy!

Ingredients:
2 cans chickpeas, drained and rinsed
½ cup hot water
¼ cup + 2 tablespoons olive oil
1 garlic clove, minced
2 tablespoons tahini
1 ½ tablespoons lemon juice
1 tablespoon lemon zest
½ teaspoon crushed red pepper
¼ teaspoon cumin

Directions:
1. Place the chickpeas, olive oil, garlic, tahini, lemon juice, lemon zest, crushed red pepper, and cumin in a food processor and pulse until smooth.
2. After 30 seconds of pulsing, pour in a little bit of hot water and continue pulsing.
3. Repeat step 2 until your hummus reaches a desired consistency.
4. Transfer your smooth and creamy hummus to an air-tight container.
5. Store hummus in the fridge overnight to let the flavors pull through.
6. Dip, dollop, snack, and enjoy!

Nutrient Breakdown (per one tablespoon):
Calories – 47
Fat in grams – 3
Carbs in grams – 4
Fiber in grams – 1
Protein in grams – 1

# Refreshing Tzatziki Sauce (makes about 3 cups)

This is always a favorite dish in the summer thanks to its light and refreshing characteristics, and it can be spread on everything from crackers to fish to veggies. I hope you enjoy this recipe just as much as I do!

Ingredients:
2 cups plain yoghurt, low fat
2 cucumbers, shredded
3 garlic cloves, minced
2 tablespoons olive oil
1 ½ tablespoons lemon juice
1 tablespoon dill, chopped
Dash of pepper

Directions:
1. Place the yoghurt in a coffee filter lined strainer and place it in the fridge for an hour to let the excess liquid drain off. Tip: Be sure to secure this contraption over a bowl or container to catch the excess liquid.
2. Once the yoghurt is drained, put it in a food processor along with the cucumber, garlic, olive oil, lemon juice, dill, and pepper.
3. Pulse ingredients until smooth and well combined.
4. Transfer your tzatziki to an air-tight container and store in the fridge overnight to let the flavors pull through.
5. Dip, dollop, snack, dress, and enjoy!

Nutrient Breakdown (per one tablespoon):
Calories – 11
Fat in grams – 1
Carbs in grams – 1
Fiber in grams – 0
Protein in grams – 1

# Traditional Mediterranean Aioli (makes about 2 cups)

In the simplest of terms, aioli is just a mayonnaise-like paste seasoned with garlic. Needless to say, it tastes amazing on pretty much everything from toast to veggies to meat. This one in particular has a creamy cashew flavor to it, which makes it much more savory than the others.

Ingredients:
1 cup cashews, soaked
½ cup water
2 garlic cloves, minced
3 tablespoons lemon juice
1 tablespoon lemon zest
1 teaspoon apple cider vinegar

Directions:
1. Drain the cashews and put them in a food processor along with the water, garlic, lemon juice, lemon zest, and apple cider vinegar.
2. Pulse ingredients until sauce is smooth and all lumps are removed.
3. Give the sauce a taste and season with extra lemon juice or pepper – whatever else you think it needs! If you do end up adding extra ingredients, just give it a couple more pulses.
4. Transfer the sauce to an air-tight container, store in the fridge, and use as needed.

Nutrient Breakdown (per one tablespoon):
Calories – 24
Fat in grams – 2
Carbs in grams – 1
Fiber in grams – 0
Protein in grams – 1

# Lemon Caper Sauce (makes about 2 cups)

The people of the Mediterranean region have been enjoying capers since the beginning of time – they grow all over the area. This is another sauce that goes great with just about anything, but let me tell you, nothing compares to the way it tastes on chicken and salmon.

Ingredients:
1 cup mayo
2 tablespoons Dijon
2 tablespoons capers, minced
1 tablespoon lemon juice
1 teaspoon parsley
½ teaspoon garlic powder
Dash of pepper

Directions:
1. Put the mayo, Dijon, capers, lemon juice, parsley, garlic powder, and pepper in a small bowl and mix together until well combined.
2. Transfer sauce to an air-tight container and store in the refrigerator.
3. Drizzle, dip, dollop, spread, and enjoy!

Nutrient Breakdown (per one tablespoon):
Calories – 29
Fat in grams – 3
Carbs in grams – 2
Fiber in grams – 0
Protein in grams – 0

# Mediterranean-Style Salsa (makes about 2 cups)

Salsa is a staple in every kitchen, which is exactly why I created a Mediterranean version for you! This one in particular is reminiscent of Greek salad, and goes great with both crackers and chicken. If you're looking to add a bright and zesty twist to your dinner, look no further than this little number!

Ingredients:
2 cups cherry tomatoes, diced
½ cup black olives, pitted and diced
½ cup feta cheese, crumbled
½ cup cucumber, diced
¼ cup red onion, diced
3 tablespoons lemon juice
1 tablespoon oregano, minced
1 tablespoon red wine vinegar
1 teaspoon paprika
Dash of pepper

Directions:
1. Put the cherry tomatoes, black olives, feta cheese, cucumber, red onion, lemon juice, oregano, red wine vinegar, paprika, and pepper in a medium-sized bowl.
2. Gently mix the ingredients together until well combined.
3. Dip, dollop, spread, and enjoy!

Nutrient Breakdown (per one tablespoon):
Calories – 9
Fat in grams – 1
Carbs in grams – 1
Fiber in grams – 0
Protein in grams – 0

## Dill Crazy Tartar Sauce (makes 2 ½ cups)

The people in the Mediterranean region love their seafood, and so they've perfected the art of creamy, delicious tartar sauce. This one puts emphasis on dill flavors, which will give your seafood dishes a refreshing twist you never thought possible!

Ingredients:
1 ¼ cups plain yoghurt, fat-free
2/3 cup mayo

¼ cup + 2 tablespoons dill pickle relish
¼ cup capers, drained and minced
1 teaspoon dill weed
½ teaspoon Italian seasoning

Directions:
1. Place the plain yoghurt, dill pickle relish, capers, dill weed, and Italian seasoning in a medium-sized bowl.
2. Mix together until well combined.
3. Transfer to an air-tight container and store in the refrigerator overnight to let flavors pull through.
4. Serve with your favorite seafood dishes to pump up the flavor and give it a new dimension!

Nutrient Breakdown (per one tablespoon):
Calories – 18
Fat in grams – 1
Carbs in grams – 1
Fiber in grams – 0
Protein in grams – 0

## Potato Skordalia (makes 1 cup)

This garlic-flavored puree from Greece goes wonderfully slathered over whole wheat rustic toast or meat. Made with simple ingredients found in any grocery store, you'll have it whipped up and ready to go in no time!

Ingredients:
½ cup olive oil
1 small russet potato, peeled and diced
4 garlic cloves, minced
2 ½ tablespoons almonds, blanched and ground
½ tablespoon red wine vinegar

Directions:
1. Put the potato in a small pot and fill with water until there is 1 inch over the potato.

2. Put the pot over high heat and let the potato boil for about 15 minutes or until soft.
3. Once the potato is soft, drain off the water and transfer to a bowl.
4. Mash with a potato masher until all lumps have been removed.
5. Once all the lumps are removed add in the garlic and almonds, stirring until well combined.
6. Once the garlic and almonds are well combined, stir in the oil and red wine vinegar until evenly distributed.
7. Transfer the mixture to an air-tight container and store in the fridge, using as needed, for the next 4 days.

Nutrient Breakdown (per one tablespoon):
Calories – 74
Fat in grams – 7
Carbs in grams –0
Fiber in grams – 0
Protein in grams – 0

# Versatile Pesto (makes about 1 cup)

As the title reads, I *love* pesto because it is just so versatile! Spread this one over crackers, whole wheat toast, or stir it into soups and pasta to add savory, refreshing, unexpected flavor. While this can be bought in store, I definitely prefer this simple homemade version. It's flavor-filled yet chemical and preservative free!

Ingredients:
3 cups basil leaves, packed
1/3 cup parmesan cheese, shredded
2 cloves garlic, minced
3 tablespoons olive oil
1 ½ tablespoons pine nuts, lightly toasted
Dash of pepper

Directions:

1. Pulse the basil leaves, parmesan cheese, garlic, pine nuts, and half of the olive oil in a food processor or blender until smooth.
2. Once mixture is smooth, add the pepper and drizzle in the rest of the olive oil, pulsing again until well incorporated.
3. Transfer to an air-tight container or jar or serve immediately. This recipe will keep in the fridge for up to 48 hours.

Nutrient Breakdown (per one tablespoon):
Calories – 14
Fat in grams – 1
Carbs in grams – 0
Fiber in grams – 0
Protein in grams – 1

## Tapenade (makes 2 cups)

I can remember making tapenade with my mother as a little girl with a can of olives pulled from the back of the pantry. I couldn't have been older than 5 years old, so needless to say, the salty flavor was a little overpowering for my tiny taste buds. I did grow to like it more the older I got, and I now bring this recipe to almost every get together I go to. It's a real hit at fancy adult parties!

Ingredients:
10 oil-packed anchovy filets, drained
1 ½ cups black olives, pitted
1 cup olive oil
½ cup capers, soaked and drained
¼ cup + 2 tablespoons almonds, sliced
4 garlic cloves, diced
2 tablespoons lemon juice

Directions:

1. Pulse the anchovy filets, black olives, capers, almonds, garlic, and a ¼ cup of the olive oil in a food processor or blender until all ingredients are chopped up.
2. Once all ingredients are chopped up, transfer the mixture to a bowl and pour in the lemon juice and remaining olive oil, stirring until all ingredients are thoroughly distributed.
3. Cover the bowl with a lid or some plastic wrap and stick it in the fridge overnight so that the flavors pull through.
4. Uncover and enjoy as needed for the next 4 days!

Nutrient Breakdown (per one tablespoon):
Calories – 75
Fat in grams – 8
Carbs in grams – 1
Fiber in grams – 0
Protein in grams – 1

# Spicy Cilantro Sauce (makes about 1 cup)

This zesty, creamy sauce goes great over pasta or shrimp. The garlic flavor is quite present yet not overwhelming, while the hot sauce and cilantro add refreshing, unexpected dynamic.

Ingredients:
1 head of garlic, top removed
1 cup cilantro leaves, minced
¼ cup olive oil
2 tablespoons lime juice
1 tablespoon white wine (dry is best)
1 tablespoon hot sauce

Directions:
1. Preheat oven to 400 degrees Fahrenheit.
2. Drizzle 1 tablespoon olive oil over the head of garlic and stick it in the oven for 10-15 minutes or until fragrant.

3. Remove the garlic from the oven and once it has cooled a bit, remove the peel and crush it down until it's a mush.
4. Transfer the mushed garlic into a bowl and add the cilantro, remaining olive oil, lime juice, white wine, and hot sauce. Mix these ingredients together until well combined.
5. Transfer to a bowl or air-tight container, store in the fridge, and serve as needed. This sauce should keep for up to 3 days.

Nutrient Breakdown (per one tablespoon):
Calories – 34
Fat in grams – 3
Carbs in grams – 1
Fiber in grams – 0
Protein in grams – 0

# Creamy Dill Sauce (makes about 2 cups)

This creamy dill sauce goes wonderfully with chicken and shrimp, or even as a pasta sauce. The low-fat Greek yoghurt is what makes it so irresistibly thick and creamy, so you don't have to worry about eating it in strict moderation. Dip, dollop, and indulge away!

Ingredients:
1 ¼ cup Greek yoghurt, low-fat
1 cup dill, stems removed and minced
1 garlic cloves, minced
1 tablespoon lime juice
1 tablespoon olive oil
Dash of hot sauce
Dash of pepper

Directions:
1. Put the Greek yoghurt, dill, garlic, lime juice, olive oil, hot sauce, and pepper in a food processor and pulse until smooth and well combined.

2. Transfer sauce to an air-tight container or bowl, depending on whether you'd like to serve it now or later.
3. Dip, dollop, savor, and enjoy! This sauce should keep in the fridge to be used as needed for up to 48 hours.

Nutrient Breakdown (per one tablespoon):
Calories – 19
Fat in grams – 1
Carbs in grams – 2
Fiber in grams – 0
Protein in grams – 1

## Greek Vinaigrette (makes 1 cup)

You didn't think I'd write a Mediterranean cookbook without a recipe for Greek salad dressing, now did you? This vinaigrette in particular has the perfect balance of lemon, garlic, and oregano flavor. I personally find myself drizzling it over green salads, quinoa salads, and pasta salads, but it goes great with pretty much anything!

Ingredients:
½ cup olive oil
½ cup lemon juice
¼ cup red wine vinegar
4 garlic cloves, minced
2 teaspoons dried oregano
½ teaspoon pepper

Directions:
1. Put the olive oil, lemon juice, red wine vinegar, garlic cloves, dried oregano, and pepper in a jar and shake it up until all ingredients are well combined.
2. Pour over salads or whatever else you think it might taste good on and enjoy! This recipe can be stored in the fridge for up to one week.

Nutrient Breakdown (per one tablespoon):

Calories – 59
Fat in grams – 6
Carbs in grams – 1
Fiber in grams – 0
Protein in grams – 0

# Chapter 9 – Seaside Sippers

## Raspberry Fig Punch (makes 4 servings)

This refreshing drink is wonderful in the spring and summer seasons. I'll often multiply the recipe to bring it to backyard parties, campfires, and BBQ's. It's a hit every time!

Main Ingredients:
¼ cup raspberry simple syrup
12 raspberries
2 figs, sliced thin
Chilled prosecco

Raspberry Syrup Ingredients:
2 tablespoons caster sugar
2 tablespoons water
2 tablespoons raspberries, crushed

Directions:
1.  Start by preparing your raspberry syrup. Place the caster sugar, water, and crushed raspberries in a saucepan and stir together.
2.  Place the saucepan over medium-low heat and keep stirring until the sugar dissolves. Then, let it sit to simmer for 2-3 minutes or until thick.
3.  Pour the syrup into a jar over a strainer to catch the pulp. Discard of the pulp.
4.  Line up four tall glasses and place a little over 1 tablespoon of syrup in each.
5.  Divide the raspberries and figs between the glasses and fill the rest of the way with prosecco.
6.  Sip, savor, and enjoy!

Nutrient Breakdown (per one serving):
Calories – 78
Fat in grams – 1
Carbs in grams – 19

Fiber in grams – 5
Protein in grams – 1

## Citrus Sangria (makes 4 servings)

This citrus sangria is perfect for girl's night in or even Tuesday
night, you know, if it's been one of those days. The citrus flavor
is light and refreshing, and the drink has a nice sweetness to it
overall.

Ingredients:
½ bottle dry white wine
½ cup sparkling water
¼ cup apricot nectar
½ lime, cut into wedges
½ orange, cut into wedges
½ lemon, cut into wedges
2 tablespoons brandy
2 tablespoons orange liqueur
2 tablespoons caster sugar
Mint leaves to garnish

Directions:
1. Put the dry white wine, apricot nectar, brandy, orange liqueur, and caster sugar in a pitcher. Stir ingredients together with a wooden spoon until sugar has dissolved.
2. Plop your fruit wedges into the pitcher and give it another quick stir.
3. Place the pitcher in the fridge to chill for at least 3 hours.
4. Once chilled, remove pitcher from the fridge, divide it between 4 glasses, and garnish each with a couple mint leaves
5. Sip, savor, and enjoy!

Nutrient Breakdown (per one serving):
Calories – 187
Fat in grams – 0
Carbs in grams – 14

Fiber in grams – 1
Protein in grams – 0

## Raspberry Mojito with an Italian Twist (makes 4 servings)

The Italian twist is in the prosecco. Other than that, this is your typical, pretty in pink, fruit flavored mojito! Sweetened with agave instead of sugar, you don't have to worry too much about your waistline with this one.

Ingredients:
24 ounces raspberries
32 mint leaves
¼ cup agave
8 ounces prosecco
8 ounces lime juice
6 ounces white rum
Ice

Directions:
1. Take 12 raspberries and 8 mint leaves and set them aside as garnish.
2. Put the remaining raspberries, mint, agave, and lime juice in a pitcher and crush with a wooden spoon or potato masher.
3. Add in the rum and stir until well combined.
4. Once the rum is well combined, stir in the prosecco until all ingredients are thoroughly distributed.
5. Pour mixture through a strainer and discard of all the bits it catches.
6. Divide the mixture between 4 glasses and garnish with the raspberry and mint you set aside at the beginning.
7. Sip, savor, and enjoy!

Nutrient Breakdown (per 1 serving):
Calories –262
Fat in grams – 1
Carbs in grams – 32

Fiber in grams – 13
Protein in grams – 3

## Waterberry Sangria (makes 4 servings)

Watermelon and strawberries come together to create a sangria both tart and sweet. Don't skip out on that garnish! The nutmeg really adds some amazing dimension to this one.

Ingredients:
325ml dry white wine
½ cup cantaloupe, diced
½ cup strawberries, sliced
½ small lemon, sliced
1 ounce orange liqueur
1 ounce Aperol
2 tablespoons honey
Nutmeg to garnish

Directions:
1. In a large pitcher, stir together the dry white wine, orange liqueur, Aperol, and honey until well combined.
2. Once the liquids are well combined, add the strawberry and cantaloupe.
3. Crush the strawberry and cantaloupe at the bottom of the pitcher with a wooden spoon or potato masher.
4. Garnish with the lemon slices and nutmeg.
5. Place the pitcher in the fridge and let it chill for a couple of hours before serving.
6. Sip, savor, and enjoy!

Nutrient Breakdown (per 1 serving):
Calories – 147
Fat in grams – 0
Carbs in grams – 16
Fiber in grams – 1
Protein in grams – 0

## Lemonade Spritzer (makes 4 servings)

This is refreshing sparkling lemonade fit for the whole family to enjoy! It's got a twist of pineapple laced through it which makes for some interesting punch and flavor. I imagine it would be great garnished with cinnamon and extra berries.

Ingredients:
½ litre sparkling water
¾ cup pineapple juice
¼ cup caster sugar
2 slices lemon
2 tablespoons honey
2 tablespoons lemon juice
Ice

Directions:
1. Put the pineapple juice, caster sugar, honey, and lemon juice in a saucepan over medium heat.
2. Bring the mixture to a boil and once it becomes a syrupy-consistency, remove it from the heat. Set aside to cool.
3. Once the syrup has cooled, fill 4 tall glasses 1/3 of the way with ice.
4. Place the lemon slices on top of the ice and drizzle the syrup over it, dividing evenly as you go.
5. Fill the glasses the rest of the way with sparkling water, serve, and enjoy!

Nutrient Breakdown (per one serving):
Calories – 110
Fat in grams – 0
Carbs in grams – 30
Fiber in grams – 1
Protein in grams – 0

## The Pink Lady (makes 4 servings)

A classy drink for all the girly girls and men who are comfortable with their masculinity, ha-ha! The lemon zest in this one adds some great color and flavor, while the egg white makes the drink nice and frothy.

Ingredients:
4 strips lemon zest
1 egg white
1 ½ ounces gin
½ ounce lemon juice
½ ounce cointreau
¼ ounce Campari
¼ ounce limoncello
Ice, crushed

Directions:
1. Put the egg white, gin, lemon juice, Cointreau, Campari, and limoncello in a cocktail shaker or jar and shake until ingredients are well combined.
2. Add the ice and shake again.
3. Pour out into 4 glasses, garnish each with a lemon zest strip, and enjoy!

Nutrient Breakdown (per one serving):
Calories – 50
Fat in grams – 0
Carbs in grams – 3
Fiber in grams – 0
Protein in grams – 1

## Olive Devil (makes 4 servings)

A drink for those who like their alcohol one way and one way only – left the way it is! Pour this into a martini glass and let the olives sink to the bottom to create a drink which looks interesting and tastes great.

Ingredients:
8 ounces white rum
4 ounces dry vermouth
4 black olives

Ice

Directions:
1. Prepare your glasses by placing them in the freezer to chill.
2. Put the white rum and dry vermouth in a cocktail shaker or jar and shake until well combined.
3. Fill the cocktail shaker halfway with ice and shake again.
4. Pour the mixture into your chilled glasses and garnish with an olive.
5. Serve and enjoy!

Nutrient Breakdown (per 1 serving):
Calories – 167
Fat in grams – 1
Carbs in grams – 1
Fiber in grams – 0
Protein in grams – 0

## Rose Petal Punch (makes 12 servings)

The first time I saw this punch was at a wedding. The venue was accented with deep purples and light pinks and this punch was almost more admired than the dang cake was! Plus, it tasted great. Upon asking the caterers about the recipe, I was quite pleasantly surprised to find that not only was it healthy, but also Mediterranean. I hope you enjoy this one as much as I do!

Ingredients:
32 ounces raspberry-apple juice, no sugar added
1 liter soda water
1 cup raspberries
120ml rose petal syrup
18 ice cubes
An edible rose for garnish

Directions:

1. Pour the raspberry-apple juice and soda water into a punch bowl.
2. Drizzle in the syrup, stirring it in until evenly distributed.
3. Place the punch in the fridge for a couple of hours to let it chill and allow the flavors to pull through.
4. When it's chilled and ready to serve, stir in the ice and top it with the raspberries and edible rose.
5. Enjoy!

Nutrient Breakdown (per 1 serving):
Calories – 52
Fat in grams – 0
Carbs in grams – 12
Fiber in grams – 1
Protein in grams – 0

# Mediterranean Adult Nestea (makes 4 servings)

It's our favorite childhood drink slightly altered to suit our adult needs! I've paired this drink with some sparkling water to give it a bit of tang and bite. It's also been paired with lots of alcohol... for those long summer nights spent with good friends.

Ingredients:
4 ounces liqueur
4 ounces orange liqueur
4 ounces orange juice
4 ounces lime juice
4 ounces syrup
Sparkling water to fill

Directions:
1. Put the liqueur, orange liqueur, orange juice, lime juice, syrup, and soda in a cocktail shaker or jar and shake until ingredients are well combined.

2. Strain the mixture and discard of any bits the strainer catches.
3. Pour into 4 glasses, dividing the mixture evenly as you go.
4. Fill the glasses the rest of the way with sparkling water.
5. Serve and enjoy!

Nutrient Breakdown (per one serving):
Calories – 216
Fat in grams – 0
Carbs in grams – 24
Fiber in grams – 0
Protein in grams – 0

## Mediterranean Twisted Coffee (makes 4 servings)

I'm a bit of a coffee freak, so, when I learned that coffee could be made with a Mediterranean twist I just couldn't *wait* to try it! This one is both sweet and spiced, and my parents always ask me to whip some up when I go to visit them. Feel free to pair it with cream or milk if that's what you usually take. However, be careful with the amount of sugar you add as this recipe already calls for a decent amount.

Ingredients:
4 cups coffee, made strong
2 ½ tablespoons caster sugar
1 teaspoon cloves
1 cinnamon stick
Dash of anise seed

Directions:
1. Put the coffee, caster sugar, cloves, cinnamon, and anise seed in a pot over medium heat.
2. Stir together until all ingredients are well combined.
3. Once the mixture reaches a temperature of 200 degrees Fahrenheit, remove it from heat.
4. Strain the mixture.

5.  Divide the mixture between four mugs, serve, and enjoy!

Nutrient Breakdown (per one serving):
Calories – 32
Fat in grams – 0
Carbs in grams – 10
Fiber in grams – 0
Protein in grams – 0

# Chapter 10 – Delicious Desserts

## Walnut Crescent Cookies (makes about 20 cookies)

I come from a German background, yet still have very fond memories of baking these Mediterranean desserts with my mother from the time I was a little girl. At first bite, they're airy like a shortbread cookie. As you keep chewing, however, a wonderful nutty flavor comes out of the woodwork. Feel free to experiment with different types of fillings. This one just happens to be my personal favorite!

Dough Ingredients:
2 cups whole wheat flour
1 cup corn oil
½ cup dry white wine
¼ cup brown sugar

Filling Ingredients:
1 cup walnuts, diced
1 apple, shredded
2 tablespoons sugar
2 tablespoons whole wheat bread crumbs
1 tablespoon strawberry jam
½ teaspoon cinnamon
Icing sugar for garnish

Directions:
1. Put the corn oil and brown sugar in a large bowl and stir together until well combined.
2. Once well combined, add the dry white wine and whole wheat flour. Beat this in until a dough forms.
3. Once a dough forms, remove it from the bowl and knead it over a flat surface until soft, but not sticky. Then, let the dough sit for 30 minutes.

4. While the dough sits, you can begin to prepare the filling. Start by putting the walnuts, apple, sugar, whole wheat bread crumbs, strawberry jam, and cinnamon in a large bowl.
5. Mix all the ingredients together until well combined. Set aside.
6. Preheat oven to 350 degrees Fahrenheit.
7. Once a half hour has passed, flatten the dough out over a floured flat surface until it is 1/5 of an inch thick.
8. Using a glass cup, cut circles out of the dough.
9. Set the circles aside, roll the remaining dough out again and repeat step 7 until little or no dough is left.
10. Once all of your dough has been cut into circles, divide the filling between them, dolloping a little bit in the center of each.
11. Fold each circle in half over top of the filling and squish the edges nicely into one another so that none of the filling can seep out.
12. Line a baking sheet with parchment paper and spread the crescents out over top.
13. Place the baking sheet in the oven and let the crescents bake for 20 minutes.
14. After 20 minutes, remove the baking sheet from the oven and sprinkle the icing sugar over top.
15. Serve and enjoy!

Nutrient Breakdown (per one crescent cookie):
Calories – 200
Fat in grams – 16
Carbs in grams – 23
Fiber in grams – 3
Protein in grams – 4

# Traditional Ekmek Kataifi (makes 12 servings)

Kataifi is one of the most popular desserts in all of Greece. Its angel hair texture is truly unique, while the nut flavors work to compliment it perfectly. This one in particular has a certain lemon flavor which makes it stand apart from the rest.

Pastry Ingredients:
1 cup kataifi dough
1/3 cup pistachios, diced
½ cup butter, melted

Syrup Ingredients:
¾ cup water
¾ cup caster sugar
1 cinnamon stick
½ tablespoon lemon zest

Custard Ingredients:
3 cups milk, cold
2/3 cup sugar
1/3 cup butter
1/3 cup corn starch
4 egg yolks
½ teaspoon vanilla extract

Directions:
1. Preheat oven to 340 degrees Fahrenheit.
2. Knead the kataifi dough, spreading apart the clumped together strands in order to create a more fluffy consistency.
3. Spray a baking dish with cooking spray and press the kataifi dough into the bottom of it, forming one even layer.
4. Pour the melted butter over top and place the baking dish in the oven for 30-40 minutes, or until it begins to turn a light brown.
5. While the kataifi is in the oven, you can begin to prepare your custard. Start by placing half of the sugar and all of the egg yolks in a bowl and whisking them together until well combined and bubbly. Then, set the mixture aside for later.

6. In a separate bowl, whisk together 4 tablespoons of milk and all of the corn starch until well combined. Set this mixture aside for later as well.
7. Pour the remaining milk into a large non-stick pan over high heat along with the sugar and vanilla extract. Stir this together well and bring the mixture to a boil.
8. Remove the pan from heat as soon as the milk begins to boil. Set aside.
9. Pour 1/3 of the pan's mixture into the egg yolk mixture and whisk it in until well combined.
10. Transfer the egg yolk mixture back into the pan and place the pan back over heat, but this time on medium.
11. Whisk continuously as this cooks, until the mixture becomes all qualities of thick, smooth, and creamy.
12. Once the mixture is thick, smooth, and deliciously creamy, remove it again from the heat.
13. Add the butter into the pan and stir it into the mixture until melted and well combined.
14. Transfer this mixture into a baking tray and place some plastic wrap over top of it. Tip: The plastic wrap should be touching the mixture to ensure it stays creamy.
15. Set this aside, let it cool, and while you're going strong, begin to prepare the syrup.
16. Stir the water, sugar, lemon zest, and cinnamon stick together in a small pot or saucepan over medium heat until the sugar has dissolved.
17. Bring the mixture to a boil and let it boil for 3 minutes until it thickens up into syrup consistency.
18. Once it's thick enough, remove it from the heat and let it cool down until it's just warm enough for you to eat it without burning your mouth.
19. By now your kataifi dough should have been removed from the oven and cooled. If this is not the case, wait until it is cool.
20. Once the kataifi is cool, ladle the syrup over top one at a time, giving each spoonful enough time to be absorbed. Then, set it aside to cool completely.
21. Once it has cooled completely, spread the creamy custard overtop of the kataifi in a nice, even layer.

22. Sprinkle the chopped pistachios over the entire thing. You can be as creative as you like! Make a smiley face or a rainbow to impress your friends...
23. Slice into 12 pieces, serve, and enjoy!

Nutrient Breakdown (per one serving):
Calories – 305
Fat in grams – 17
Carbs in grams – 35
Fiber in grams – 1
Protein in grams – 5

## Flaky Coconut Pie (makes 8 servings)

This one is light and flaky with a delectable coconut flavor to keep you coming back for more. You could top this one with fresh fruit to add a little more color and nutrition, but it's wonderful on its own as well.

Ingredients:
11 sheets filo pastry
400 ml coconut cream
½ cup cashews, chopped
½ cup caster sugar
¼ cup butter, melted
¼ cup shredded coconut, unsweetened
2 eggs
1 teaspoon vanilla extract
Icing sugar to garnish

Directions:
1. Preheat oven to 350 degrees Fahrenheit.
2. Grease a pie dish with just enough melted butter to cover it.
3. In a medium size bowl, whisk together the coconut cream, caster sugar, eggs and vanilla until all ingredients are well combined and the sugar has to dissolve. Set this aside for later.

4. Pulse the cashews and shredded coconut in a food processor until it turns into mulch. Set this aside as well.
5. Place a piece of the filo pastry on a clean, stable surface and brush a generous amount of butter over it.
6. Roughly scrunch the piece of filo pastry up and place it in the pie dish.
7. Repeat steps 5-6 until the baking tray is full.
8. Once your pie dish is full, pour the coconut cream mixture over top, making sure each inch of the pastry gets soaked in it.
9. Once you're out of your coconut cream mixture, sprinkle the cashew mixture over top.
10. Place the pie dish in the oven and let it bake for 25-35 minutes or until the top has turned a nice golden-brown and the pastry has risen.
11. Remove the baking tray from the oven and allow your pie to cool for 15 minutes.
12. Sprinkle the icing sugar over top, slice into 8 wedges, and enjoy!

Nutrient Breakdown (per one serving):
Calories – 388
Fat in grams – 25
Carbs in grams – 36
Fiber in grams – 1
Protein in grams – 6

## Ricotta Cheese Fruit Bake (makes 6 servings)

Make sure you start this recipe a day before you need it as the ricotta cheese needs to drain overnight! The time spent waiting is *so* worth it though. It's creamy, sweet qualities will have you singing songs of love at first bite!

Ricotta Cheese Ingredients:
1 ½ cups ricotta cheese
1 egg
3 tablespoons honey

1 teaspoon lemon zest

Fruit Syrup Ingredients:
1 cup cherries, pits removed and diced
3 tablespoons caster sugar
2 tablespoons orange juice
1 teaspoon orange blossom water

Directions:
1. Place ricotta cheese in a coffee filter-lined strainer and place this in the fridge to drain overnight. Tip: Make sure you place this contraption over a container so that the drained liquid won't spill everywhere!
2. Once your ricotta cheese has drained, preheat the oven to 400 degrees Fahrenheit.
3. Spray down 6 small heat-proof bowls with cooking spray.
4. Place the drained ricotta, egg, honey, and lemon in a bowl and beat this together until well combined.
5. Divide the ricotta mixture between your 6 greased bowls and place them in the oven for 30-35 minutes, or until they have turned a nice golden-brown color.
6. Once they have turned a nice golden-brown color, remove them from the oven and let them cool.
7. While your ricotta cheese bowls are cooling, you can begin to prepare the fruit sauce. Start by placing the cherries, caster sugar, and orange juice in a small pot or saucepan over medium-high heat. Stir as it reaches a boil so that ingredients are well combined and the sugar dissolves.
8. Once the mixture is boiling reduce the heat to medium-low and continue to cook, stirring occasionally, for 20-25 minutes or until the cherries are tender and the mixture takes on a syrupy consistency.
9. Once the mixture is syrupy, remove it from the heat and stir in the orange blossom water until well combined. Then, let the mixture cool a little.
10. Once the ricotta cheese bowls have cooled, divide the fruit syrup over them.

11. Serve and enjoy!

Nutrient Breakdown (per one serving):
Calories – 153
Fat in grams – 6
Carbs in grams – 21
Fiber in grams – 1
Protein in grams – 6

# Anginetti Lemon Cookies (makes 12 cookies)

These cookies are best known across southern Italy where they can be found in coffee and doughnut cafes on the daily. This recipe in particular gives them a lemon twist so fresh and irresistible you won't be able to resist!

Cookie Ingredients:
2/3 cup whole wheat flour
1 egg
2 ½ tablespoons sugar
2 tablespoons unsalted butter, warm
2/3 teaspoon baking powder
2/3 teaspoon vanilla extract
1/3 teaspoon grated lemon zest

Icing Ingredients:
1 cup powdered sugar, sifted
2 teaspoons lemon juice
2 teaspoons water
1 teaspoon butter
1/3 teaspoon vanilla extract

Directions:
1. Preheat oven to 350 degrees Fahrenheit.
2. Prepare a baking sheet by lining it with foil.
3. Start with the cookies. Beat the sugar, unsalted butter, vanilla extract, and lemon zest together until ingredients are well combined.

4. Once ingredients are well combined, crack the egg into the mixture and beat it in as well. Then, set this mixture aside for later.
5. In a separate bowl, stir together the whole wheat flour and baking powder until well combined.
6. Gradually add this to the wet mixture, beating it in as you go.
7. Once your cookie dough is smooth and lump-free, begin to dollop it out onto the lined baking sheet. You should be able to get 12 cookies out of the mixture.
8. Place the baking sheet into the oven and bake for 10-12 minutes or until they become a nice golden-brown color.
9. While the cookies are in the oven, you can begin to prepare the icing. Start by putting the butter in a small pot or saucepan over medium heat.
10. Once the butter has melted, add in the sugar, lemon juice, water, and vanilla extract, stirring ingredients into the butter until well combined. Tip: If the icing seems to be a bit thick, add a little more water to thin it out.
11. Once the cookies are done, brush the lemon icing over top while they're still hot.
12. After you've applied the icing, let the cookies sit to cool.
13. Once the cookies are cool, feel free to dig in!

Nutrient Breakdown (per one cookie):
Calories – 91
Fat in grams – 3
Carbs in grams – 15
Fiber in grams – 1
Protein in grams – 1

# Toasted Almond Biscotti (makes 20 biscotti's)

Biscotti's are a staple in any Italian household, and this recipe ensures that no matter what your health goals are, it can stay that way! I like to experiment by coating them with different seeds, nuts, or even dried fruit, but over the years found that sesame seeds taste the best.

Ingredients:
1 ¼ cups whole wheat flour
½ cup sugar
1/3 cup almonds, toasted and chopped
½ stick unsalted butter, melted
2 small eggs
1 small egg beaten with ½ tablespoon water
2 ½ tablespoons sesame seeds, toasted
1 tablespoon orange flower water
1 teaspoon anise seeds
¾ teaspoon baking powder
½ teaspoon vanilla extract
¼ teaspoon almond extract

Directions:
1. In a medium-sized bowl, mix together the sugar, almonds, orange flower water, anise seeds, vanilla extract, almond extract, and 2 tablespoons sesame seeds until well combined.
2. Once all ingredients are well combined, crack the 2 eggs into the mixture and beat them in until thoroughly distributed.
3. Once eggs are thoroughly distributed, gradually beat in the flour and baking powder until a dough forms.
4. Place this dough in the fridge to cool for a half hour.
5. Once your dough is cool, preheat oven to 350 degrees Fahrenheit.
6. Coat your hands and a clean, stable surface with flour and knead the dough into a rectangular loaf.
7. Transfer this loaf to a baking sheet and brush the egg-water over it until the entire loaf is covered.
8. Once your loaf is covered in egg wash, coat the outside with your remaining sesame seeds.
9. Place the loaf in the oven and let it bake for about 15 minutes, or until it begins to turn a light-gold color.

10. Once your loaf has turned a light-gold color, take it out of the oven and transfer it to a cooling rack. Let it sit here for about 15 minutes. Tip: Don't turn the oven off! You'll need it in just a little bit...
11. Once your loaf is cool enough to touch, slice it into 20 pieces and arrange them, cut side down, on another lined baking sheet.
12. Place the baking sheet back in the oven and let the biscotti's bake for another 15-20 minutes, or until they have turned a nice golden-brown color.
13. Remove the baking pan from the oven, let the cookies cool, and enjoy with some tea or coffee!

Nutrient Breakdown (per one biscotti):
Calories – 77
Fat in grams – 4
Carbs in grams – 10
Fiber in grams – 1
Protein in grams – 2

## Greek Rice Pudding (makes 2 servings)

This dessert is amazing both warm or cold, although it is traditionally served chilled. Finish it off with a sprinkle of cinnamon or a couple berries to create a dish that's truly indulgent and eye-catching.

Ingredients:
2 1/3 cups full-fat milk
3 tablespoons rice
3 tablespoons caster sugar
½ tablespoon corn flour
1 teaspoon cold water

Directions:
1. Put a pot with the milk over medium-high heat and cook until it comes to a boil.
2. Once the milk comes to a boil, reduce the heat to medium-low and stir in the rice and caster sugar until

well combined. Keep stirring until the sugar is completely dissolved.

3. Once the sugar has dissolved, turn the heat down to low and let the mixture cook for 20-30 minutes, or until rice has cooked. Tip: You'll need to check on this and give it the occasional stir to ensure it doesn't burn.

4. Once the rice is cooked and tender, mix the corn flour and water together in a small bowl until a smooth yet liquidy paste forms. Use more water if needed.

5. Add the corn flour mixture to the pot and stir it in until well combined.

6. Let the pudding simmer, stirring constantly, until it reaches your desired consistency.

7. Remove from heat, divide between two bowls, and serve!

Nutrient Breakdown (per one serving):
Calories – 219
Fat in grams – 9
Carbs in grams – 27
Fiber in grams – 1
Protein in grams – 10

# Doughnut Holes (makes about 10 doughnut holes)

These are popular in coffee shops almost everywhere in the world now, but they did in fact originate in Greece. Here is a more traditional recipe, and also one that's a little more health conscious than what you buy in stores.

Ingredients:
1 ¼ cups water, room temperature
1 cup whole wheat flour
¼ cup corn starch
1 tablespoon honey
1 ½ teaspoons dry yeast
Olive oil for frying

Directions:
1. Place the water, whole wheat flour, corn starch, honey, and dry yeast in a medium-sized bowl and beat until well combined.
2. Once all ingredients are well combined, set the mixture aside to rest for a half hour.
3. Fill a medium-sized pot half-way with olive oil and put it on the stove to heat to 340 degrees Fahrenheit.
4. Fill a separate bowl with some room temperature olive oil and dip a tablespoon sized spoon into it.
5. After you've dunked a spoon in the olive oil, use it to scoop up some of the doughnut hole batter and drop it into the hot pot of oil.
6. Put 5-6 doughnut holes in the pot at a time and let fry for 1 minute or until golden-brown.
7. Once the doughnut holes are golden brown, scoop them out of the oil and place them on a cooling rack (preferably with paper towel underneath) to finish crisping.
8. Repeat steps 5-7 until all of your batter is used up.
9. Once your doughnut holes have cooled toss them in a bowl with the honey and cinnamon.
10. Serve and enjoy!

Nutrient Breakdown (per one doughnut hole):
Calories – 117
Fat in grams – 0
Carbs in grams – 12
Fiber in grams – 1
Protein in grams – 2

## Sweet Ricotta-Filled Sandwiches (makes 6 sandwiches)

Sandwiches should be their own food group, am I right? When I learned that these dessert sandwiches originated in the Mediterranean region I just couldn't wait to share them with you. This recipe is both delicious yet health conscious, so there's no reason to feel guilty after scarfing one down!

Batter Ingredients:
1 cup whole wheat flour
½ cup water, room temperature
1 small egg
2 tablespoons caster sugar
2 tablespoons lard
1 teaspoon yeast
Olive oil for frying
Icing sugar to garnish

Filling Ingredients:
1 cup ricotta cheese
¾ cup caster sugar
2 tablespoons dark chocolate chips
½ teaspoon vanilla extract

Directions:
1. Place the ricotta cheese, caster sugar, and vanilla extract in a bowl and mix until mixture is well combined and smooth.
2. Once the mixture is smooth, add the chocolate chips and stir them in until evenly distributed.
3. Transfer the mixture to the fridge and let it chill for 2 hours.
4. In the meantime, you can work on the sandwich part of this dessert. Mix together the yeast, half of the sugar, and the lukewarm water in a bowl until well combined. Then let it sit to activate.
5. While your yeast is activating, sift the flour into a large-sized bowl along with the remaining sugar and lard. Beat this together until the batter is frothy.
6. Once the batter is frothy, pour in the yeast mixture and knead the batter with your hands until it becomes dough-like.
7. As you knead, crack in the egg and pour in a little bit of water to create a thick, sticky consistency.
8. Once your batter is thick and sticky, let it sit for 1 hour in a covered, greased bowl so that it can rise.

9. Once your dough has risen, pat some flour on your hands and divide it into 6 even balls. Place these on a parchment paper-lined baking sheet and let them sit to rise for another half hour.
10. Heat a dry fryer or large pot with the oil until it reaches 340 degrees Fahrenheit.
11. Drop your dough balls into the hot oil one at a time and let them fry until they turn a golden-brown color.
12. Once your dough balls are finished fryer, place them on a surface lined with paper towel so that they can finish crisping.
13. When the dough balls are cool enough to touch, slice them in half. Now each dough ball is one sandwich.
14. Divide the ricotta cheese filling between each of your sandwiches. You should be able to put a very generous amount in each!
15. Sprinkle with icing sugar to make them look pretty.
16. Plate, serve, and enjoy!

Nutrient Breakdown (per one sandwich):
Calories – 365
Fat in grams – 18
Carbs in grams – 24
Fiber in grams – 3
Protein in grams – 9

## Sesame Seed Crackers

Think peanut brittle, but with a sesame seed twist. These are mouth-wateringly crispy and sweet, yet won't break the bank or the button off your jeans! I love to bring them to work as a midday pick-me-up or indulge in some after dinner.

Ingredients:
½ cup sesame seeds
¼ cup caster sugar
1 tablespoon honey

Directions:

1. Line a baking sheet with parchment paper.
2. Place the sesame seeds in a pan over low heat to toast them. Tip: Make sure you continuously shake or stir the sesame seeds so that they don't burn!
3. Once the sesame seeds are a light-gold color, remove them from heat.
4. Stir the caster sugar and honey together until well combined in a saucepan over medium heat. Keep stirring this mixture until the sugar dissolves and the honey comes to a boil.
5. Once the honey begins to boil, stop stirring and let it do its own thing for a little over a minute. Then, remove the mixture from heat and set aside.
6. Fold your sesame seeds into the honey mixture and mix until they're thoroughly distributed.
7. Once the sesame seeds are evenly spread throughout the honey, spread the mixture out onto the baking sheet you lined with parchment paper earlier. Tip: You have to work fast at doing this! The mixture will harden very quickly.
8. Cover the honey-sesame layer with another piece of parchment paper and very gently flatten the mixture with a rolling pin. You can make it as thick or as thin as you'd like!
9. Leave the mixture to cool a little before peeling off the parchment paper and transferring it to a cutting board.
10. Using a knife, slice the mixture into as many crackers as you'd like! Tip: This is easiest if you first coat the knife in oil.
11. Let your sesame crackers cool completely and enjoy!

Nutrient Breakdown (per 1/6 recipe):
Calories – 83
Fat in grams – 4
Carbs in grams – 19
Fiber in grams – 2
Protein in grams – 2

# Avocado & Sweet Potato Cupcakes (makes 12 cupcakes)

Here's a combination which you probably never dreamed would be so delicious... The sweet potato works to make the cupcakes incredibly moist, while the avocado creates a health conscious frosting that's irresistibly creamy. The kids will love them! Just don't tell them what they're really made of...

Batter Ingredients:
1 cup + 2 tablespoons sweet potato, mashed
1 cup whole wheat flour
¾ cup caster sugar
½ cup unsalted butter, room temperature
2 eggs
2 tablespoons brown sugar
1 teaspoon baking powder
½ teaspoon cinnamon
¼ teaspoon vanilla extract
¼ teaspoon baking soda

Frosting Ingredients:
2 avocados, mashed
½ cup agave nectar
½ cup cocoa powder
½ teaspoon vanilla extract

Directions:
1.   Preheat oven to 350 degrees Fahrenheit.
2.   Line a 12-insert cupcake tray with cupcake cups and set aside.
3.   Whisk together the whole wheat flour, baking powder, and baking soda in a medium-sized bowl until well combined. Set this aside for later.
4.   In a separate bowl, beat together the caster sugar and butter until well combined.
5.   Once the caster sugar and butter are well combined, crack in the eggs and beat them in as well.

6. Once the eggs are thoroughly distributed, dump in the mashed sweet potato and vanilla extract. Mix this in until well incorporated.
7. Add the dry mixture to the wet mixture and fold it in until well combined.
8. Scoop your cupcake batter into the inserts, dividing evenly as you go, and place the cupcake tray in the oven for 10-15 minutes or until the tops of the cupcakes are golden-brown and bouncy.
9. Remove the cupcake tray from the oven and let the cupcakes sit to cool for a couple minutes.
10. Once the cupcakes are cool enough to touch, transfer them to a cooling rack to finish cooling.
11. While the cupcakes finish cooling, you can prepare the avocado frosting. Begin by placing the mashed avocados, agave nectar, cocoa powder, and vanilla extract in a bowl.
12. Beat the frosting ingredients together until smooth and well combined. Tip: You'll know you're done when the green of the avocados is no longer visible!
13. Once the cupcakes are completely cool, spread the avocado frosting overtop, dividing it evenly as you go.
14. Plate, serve, and enjoy!

Nutrient Breakdown (per one cupcake):
Calories – 234
Fat in grams – 15
Carbs in grams – 23
Fiber in grams – 6
Protein in grams – 3

# Spanish Fartons (makes 8 servings)

These elegant, thin and flaky desserts are traditional to Valencia in particular, where the people of this region have been known to eat them with hot chocolate, coffee, tea, and even cold milk. They are light as air and have a soft, chewy inside which everyone will find a hard time passing up.

Dough Ingredients:
4 ¾ cups whole wheat flour
½ cup olive oil
½ cup water
½ cup caster sugar
2 eggs
½ tablespoon dry double active yeast

Icing Ingredients:
1 ¼ cups powdered sugar
¼ cup water, room temperature

Directions:
1. Mix the water with the yeast until the yeast dissolves.
2. Sift the flour into a large mixing bowl and add in the yeast water, caster sugar, and eggs. Beat ingredients together, adding the olive oil in as you go.
3. Once a dough-like substance forms, begin to knead it with your hands, making sure all ingredients are well combined.
4. Shape the dough into a large ball and place it in a bowl.
5. Cover this bowl with plastic wrap and leave the dough to sit for 2 hours. During this time, it should double in size.
6. Once the dough has risen, preheat the oven to 360 degrees Fahrenheit and begin to roll them out into long, breadstick-like shapes. These are your fartons.
7. Place the fartons on a baking sheet lined with parchment paper and let them bake for 15-20 minutes, or until they turn a golden-brown color.
8. While the fartons are in the oven, you can begin to prepare the glaze. Start by placing both the powdered sugar and lukewarm water in a bowl.
9. Whisk these two ingredients together until it becomes thick like syrup. Then, set it aside.
10. Once the fartons are done, remove them from the oven and brush them with the glaze while they're hot.
11. Serve with a cup of hot cocoa and enjoy!

Nutrient Breakdown (per one farton):
Calories – 503
Fat in grams – 16
Carbs in grams – 96
Fiber in grams – 9
Protein in grams – 11

# Classic Cannoli's (makes 24 cannoli's)

I remember working in an Italian bakery as a teenager that had fresh cannoli's shipped in every morning. They always smelled so great... it was hard to keep our hands off them! As I've grown up, I've learned to make them in a way which is a bit more waistline friendly, which resulted in this recipe right here.

Shell Ingredients:
1 cup almond flour
1 cup cream cheese, room temperature
1 cup vanilla whey protein
½ cup butter, melted
4 egg whites

Filling Ingredients:
1 ½ cups cream cheese
1 ½ cups ricotta cheese
½ cup Swerve
1 teaspoon vanilla
1 teaspoon cinnamon

Directions:
1.  Place the ricotta cheese in a coffee filter-lined strainer and let drain in the fridge overnight. Tip: Be sure to put this contraption over a container to catch the excess liquid!
2.  Once your ricotta cheese is drained, whip the egg whites up until they are frothy.

3. Once the egg whites are frothy, add in the almond flour, cream cheese, vanilla whey powder, and butter and beat until mixture is smooth.
4. Spray a skillet down with cooking spray and put it over high heat.
5. Once the skillet is hot, place 1 tablespoon of the egg white mixture onto it.
6. Let this cook like a mini pancake for 1-3 minutes or until light brown on one side.
7. Flip and let it cook until light brown on the other side. Then, transfer it to a plate.
8. Roll the pastry into a cylinder shape before it cools and set aside.
9. Repeat steps 5-8 until all of the egg white mixture has been used up. You should be able to get 12 cannoli shells out of the mixture.
10. After you've run out of egg white mixture, you can begin to prepare the filling. Start by placing the mascarpone cheese, ricotta cheese, swerve, ground cinnamon, and vanilla extract in a bowl.
11. Mix all of the ingredients together until well combined.
12. Once all of the ingredients are well combined, cover the bowl and let it sit in the fridge for at least 4 hours.
13. After the filling has chilled, transfer it to a Ziploc bag and cut the corner off to create a piping bag.
14. Pipe the filling into each end of each shell, letting it overflow a little bit.
15. Serve immediately or store in the fridge for up until 24 hours until you're ready to eat! Enjoy.

Nutrient Breakdown (per one cannoli):
Calories – 118
Fat in grams – 8
Carbs in grams – 2
Fiber in grams – 0
Protein in grams – 8

# Vasilopita Cake (makes 10 servings)

This Greek dish is a little different than the others as traditionally, a gold coin or other trinket is hidden inside of it for one lucky person to find. Finding the coin symbolizes good luck for an entire year, but you'll be happy whether or not you're the one who finds the coin!

Ingredients:
6 eggs
3 cups whole wheat flour
2 cups caster sugar
1 cup milk
1 cup unsalted butter, room temperature
¾ cup sliced almonds
1/3 cup brown sugar
1 tablespoon anise seed
1 tablespoon honey
2 teaspoons lemon juice
2 teaspoons baking powder
1 teaspoon vanilla extract
½ teaspoon baking soda
Optional: A chocolate coin or hard candy

Directions:
1. Preheat oven the 350 degrees Fahrenheit.
2. Spray a tiered cake pan down with cooking spray.
3. Put the almonds, brown sugar, and honey in a bowl. Stir together until ingredients are well combined and then set it aside.
4. In a separate bowl, whisk together the whole wheat flour, anise seed, baking powder, and baking soda until well combined. Set this aside as well.
5. In a large bowl, beat together the caster sugar and butter until well combined.
6. Once the caster sugar and butter are well combined, crack the eggs in one at a time and beat them in as well.
7. Once the eggs are thoroughly distributed, pour in the lemon juice and vanilla, beating again until well combined.

8. Sift the flour mixture into the butter mixture and beat the two together well.
9. Once the flour mixture and butter mixture are well combined, beat in the milk.
10. Pour 1/3 of the almond mixture into the bottom of your tiered cake pan.
11. Layer half of the batter over the almond mixture.
12. Place the cake pan in the oven and bake for 25-30 minutes, or until the batter starts to firm up.
13. Once the batter starts to firm up, remove it from the oven and pour half of the remaining almond mixture over it.
14. Plop the gold coin or candy over the almond mixture and top it with the remainder of the batter.
15. Place the cake pan bake in the oven for another 25-30 minutes, or until a fork comes out clean when pierced.
16. Remove the cake pan from the oven and let the cake cool for 10 minutes before shaking it out.
17. Top the cake with the remaining almond mixture and serve while it's warm!

Nutrient Breakdown (per one serving):
Calories – 584
Fat in grams – 27
Carbs in grams – 78
Fiber in grams – 6
Protein in grams – 10

## Honey Crisps (makes 16 crisps)

This is a great platter for feeding a crowd. The Greeks love to eat them at Christmas, but I like to make them all year round! Optionally, you can top these guys with a sprinkle of cinnamon or some chopped up nuts to add new dynamic.

Cookie Batter Ingredients:
1½ cups whole wheat flour
½ cup corn oil
¼ cup orange juice

5 eggs (whites and yolks separated)
2 tablespoons lemon juice
2 tablespoons caster sugar
2 tablespoons baking soda
1 tablespoon white wine vinegar
Olive oil for frying

Syrup Ingredients:
½ cup honey
¼ cup water
¼ cup caster sugar
1 tablespoon lemon juice
1 cinnamon stick

Directions:
1. Place the egg whites in a medium-sized bowl and beat them until white peaks begin to form.
2. Once white peaks begin to form, add the egg yolks while you continue to beat the mixture.
3. Once all of the egg yolks are well combined, stir the orange juice, lemon juice, and baking soda together in a separate bowl until the baking soda dissolves.
4. Once the baking soda dissolves, pour the mixture in with the eggs.
5. Add the white wine vinegar and caster sugar to the mix and beat again until thoroughly incorporated.
6. Sift the flour in gradually as you beat.
7. Once the mixture has formed dough, knead it with your hands until it is smooth. Tip: If the dough is sticky, add a little more flour.
8. Divide the dough into four pieces, place each in a bowl, and cover with plastic wrap. Let this sit for 30 minutes.
9. After 30 minutes, roll each piece out into a thin sheet.
10. Put the olive oil in a deep fryer or pan and heat the oil.
11. Cut the dough sheets into rectangular pieces.
12. Once the oil is hot, add about 4 rectangular dough pieces to the pot and fry. Once the bottom side is golden-brown, flip it to brown the other side.

13. Once your rectangles are brown, transfer them to a surface lined with paper towel to finish crisping.
14. Repeat steps 12 and 13 until all of the dough has been used up.
15. Begin to prepare the syrup by putting the honey, water, caster sugar, lemon juice, and cinnamon stick in a small pot or saucepan over medium-high heat. Stir while the ingredients heat up so that the sugar dissolves.
16. Once the mixture comes to a boil, let it boil for 5 minutes or until the syrup thickens.
17. Arrange the fried rectangles on a serving plate and drizzle the syrup over top of them.
18. Serve and enjoy!

Nutrient Breakdown (per one crisp)
Calories – 197
Fat in grams – 11
Carbs in grams – 22
Fiber in grams – 1
Protein in grams – 3

# Epilogue

I hope the first part of this book offered great insight to the lives of the people in the Mediterranean region – habits, health benefits, and all! While the bit focusing on studies may have been quite bland in comparison to the lively Mediterranean lifestyle, I hope it did show you why there is so much praise directed towards the diet. It has kept our people healthy for countless generations, and we know so based on the cold, hard facts presented to us in studies of the past and studies of today.

I hope this diet is the one that shows you why the rest never really worked out. The Mediterranean lifestyle is about living life to the fullest, and that's exactly what I hope it helps you do. If adhered to, the Mediterranean diet is a true miracle worker in the way of building relationships and creating memories to last a lifetime – all while you eat delicious, home-cooked meals that don't take a degree in rocket-science to put together.

At the end of the day, nothing makes my career more worthwhile than when I see people benefit personally from my advice and hard efforts. As someone who is dedicated to their career in health, nothing makes me happier than watching my clients realize their potential as they succeed in improving their lives. I wish you a lifetime of feeling good, looking good, and doing good – whether you're cutting health conscious cookies with the kids or enjoying some sangria poolside with good friends.

Making the decision to live a healthier life shouldn't hold you back from all that life has to offer, and I hope the Mediterranean diet proves to you just that.

I hope this book was able to teach you on how to implement the Mediterranean diet in your daily life.

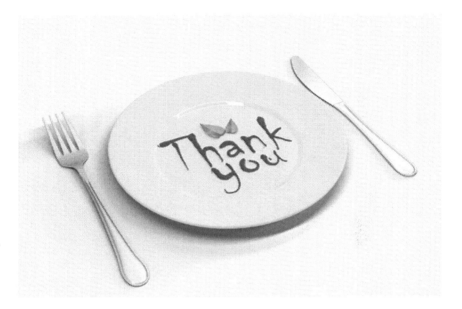

If you enjoyed this book, then I'd like to ask you for a favor, would you be kind enough to leave a review for this book on Amazon? It'd be greatly appreciated!

Also, I would love to give you a bonus. Please email me at vanessa.olsen400p@gmail.com to avail the FREE Paleo Diet book.

Please check out my other books in Amazon:
- **Ketogenic Diet** - Achieve Rapid Weight Loss while Gaining Incredible Health and Energy
- **Ketogenic Diet Cookbook** - 80 Easy, Delicious, and Healthy Recipes to Help You Lose Weight, Boost Your Energy, and Prevent Cancer, Stroke and Alzheimer's
- **Ketogenic Diet-2 in 1 Box Set** - A Complete Guide to the Ketogenic Diet-115 Amazing Recipes for Weight Loss and Improved Health

Thank you and good luck!

Made in the USA
San Bernardino, CA
09 May 2016